I Hear the Whistle Blowin'
The Final Station

A story of a family's journey
through cancer loss, and recovery.

by Judith Cyrus

Dedicated to "The Family"

To Gene

Now when the sun says good day
to the mountains
And the night says hello to the dawn
I'm alone with my dreams on the hilltop
I can still hear your voice though you're gone

I hear from my door the love songs
through the wind
It brings back sweet memories of you

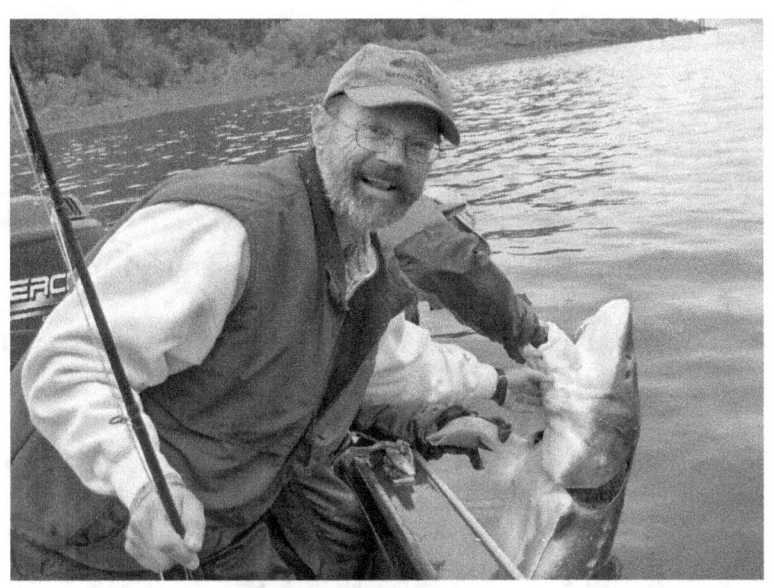

PROLOGUE

On October 2, 2006, we were casually going about our busy lives, running kids back and forth to school, building a barn, riding horses and stacking firewood. On October 3rd our lives stopped in their tracks as we became obsessed with the business of survival.

We were driving into town about 10:30 AM our second trip in after the 8:00 school run. Ellie had been home with us (Tuesdays and Thursdays are our days with our little granddaughter while Juli teaches preschool) and we were headed into town to drop her off and go up to the new barn to meet the framing contractor. Gene suddenly began moaning and holding his chest. I got him to pull over, switched sides, and drove him in to the ER, thinking he must be having a cardiac event. At the ER, they did an EKG which was normal, then did a chest Xray to see if he might have pleurisy. The

1

doctor came back and said there was a mass in Gene's lung and he wanted to do a CT scan. The hospital was in the process of opening a new wing and the brand new CT scanner was crying to be used. We kind of thought the doctor just wanted a chance to try it out. But 30 minutes later we were reading a report identifying a fist-sized mediastinal mass in Gene's left lung. The ER doctor tried to reach our family doctor so she could decide what to do, but she wasn't in so he called a surgeon and made us an appointment.

Two days later, we visited with the surgeon, who told us the mass did not really look like lung cancer because there did not seem to be any other abnormal areas in the lungs. And, since Gene has never smoked, he did not really seem at risk for lung cancer. But something clearly had to be done about the large mass, which was now causing constant pain, so he scheduled a biopsy to identify it and decide on a treatment plan. The biopsy was done on Wednesday, October 11th. We were told the results would be available in 3 to 5 days unless there were complications in reading the slides, in which case they would be sent to a larger facility for interpretation. In that case, it would take about a week.

After three days, we called the surgeon's office but the results were not in. We repeated the call every day or two for 2 weeks, with no luck.

On October 25th, about 11:30 PM I took Gene back to the ER because he was in so much pain the Vicodin no longer helped. Dr. Sherpa did an X-ray and found the mass had grown considerably so did another CT scan and sent it off for analysis. When we got back the new measurements, we found the mass had tripled in size during the three weeks since the first scan. I was horrified, and the next day we drove to The Dalles, Oregon to the surgeon's office, CT scans in hand on a CD. We asked to talk to the surgeon, hoping to get a stronger pain medication, find out why the biopsy results were still not there, and ask what could be done with this rapidly growing mass in the meantime. The nurse came out to give us a prescription and tell us the results were still not available. We began asking her why it was taking so long and what could be done in the meantime. The surgeon heard us and came out. He pushed us into an exam room and proceeded to read us the riot act for asking his staff "inappropriate questions." This made me mad and I told him we were asking her the questions because she was the only one who would talk to us so we *could* ask questions. Then I told him our pets were getting better medical care than my husband. I guess he didn't like that much and soon we were hustling out the door. I was so angry and frustrated that I drove straight to our family doctor's office to try to get some help. She was not there and the triage nurse was at lunch, so the receptionist wrote down our story, expressing shock at our treatment by the surgeon. The triage nurse called us about 30 minutes later and then spent the next couple of hours calling the pathologists to find out what was going on with the report. She also called OHSU to see if we could find an alternate path to treatment. In the end, she was in tears as she explained that the pathologists assured her the report would be sent later that day or at the latest, the following morning. She said, "I promise you that when the report is here, if it is something that needs immediate attention, Dr. Taylor will see you immediately."

Later that day, the surgeon called to tell us he had gotten the report and that Gene had large cell lung cancer. This terrifying news set us off on an emotional roller coaster that we shared with family and friends via a website called Caring Bridge (www.caringbridge.org) This book is primarily a re-creation of the journal and a few of the guest book entries from that site. However, I have since supplemented those entries with some of the additional thoughts and experiences that at the time seemed too private to post on the internet. I have added entries from my personal journal that describe my bumbling through the grief process. Some of these are very personal but my hope for this book is that others will be comforted, encouraged, or at least informed about a process they may be dumped into unexpectedly, as we were. I can't really offer any answers; I am struggling to find them myself, but I believe there is comfort in sharing burdens with others. For that reason, I feel it is necessary to go the additional step to include the rest of the story.

But first, maybe some introductions are in order.

Gene likes to tell the story about how we met. He was home from college for Christmas vacation and saw me riding by on my big appaloosa gelding. As Gene tells the story, he asked his brother who the girl was and Dennis responded, "Judi Johnson, she's cute, huh?" Gene said, "I don't know about that, but I'd sure like to ride her horse."

A little over a year later, we were married. Gene went to a year of graduate school, then in 1971 began his career with the US Forest Service. Also in 1971, our first daughter, Juli, was born. Two years later, Jaimi arrived and four years after, that, Jillian. I loved staying home to be a full time mommy but when Jill went to Kindergarten, I went to college. My last year of school, Gene was offered a job in Germany, something we had always hoped for since we both wanted to "see the world." So I finished college by correspondence then began my career with Hewlett Packard while living in Germany.

By the time Jill was in high school, my career was going well and we were starting to get angsty over the thought of an empty nest. We had a blast with our girls and couldn't really face the idea of not having kids at home to play with. We decided we wanted to adopt a couple of children. Somehow we ended up adopting a sibling group of six. This turned out to be more of a challenge than we anticipated, but that's life for you, I guess.

In 1997, we had the opportunity to go to Panama for a couple of years. While we were there, we adopted a beautiful little Panamanian who we named Kalle. About the same time, Juli and Jaimi each got married. Juli and her husband Rob have two children, Dillon and Ellie. Jaimi has a son,

Kevin, who is the same age as Dillon and his best friend, even though he lives on the other side of the world in Germany. And that completed our family, and completes the introductions you need to get started in our story.

FRIDAY, OCTOBER 27, 2006
2:04 AM

Today was our first visit to Celilo Cancer Center. It is a pretty amazing place. They treat body, mind and soul and offer a lot of services to help the whole family through a tough ordeal, in addition to treating the patient.

While we were checking in with the receptionist, she took a phone call. After talking for a few minutes, she said, "I am just checking them in now." and handed me the phone. It was Dr. Sherpa, the ER doc, who had called our house, found no one home so called the surgeon's office who told him we had been referred here. He tracked us down just to see how we were doing. I was amazed and it really lifted our spirits to find such a caring doctor.

Daughters Juli, Jill and I all went with Gene into his first meeting with Dr. Steltzer, the radiation oncologist, who spent a lot of time explaining the diagnosis and the ambiguity of it. He said the diagnosis was somewhat vague because the sample sent for the biopsy had so many dead cells in it that it was hard to read. I asked him why there would be so many dead cells, and he said that was typical of a mass growing so fast because the rapid growth caused the tumor to outgrow its blood supply and

6

cells would die off. Jill asked if that should have been a clue to the pathologists that the mass was rapidly growing and that immediate treatment was critical. Apparently though, pathologists just read slides and the diagnosis takes as long as it takes, external logic is not useful. . . Dr. Steltzer told us what he proposed for initial treatment until further tests could be done to customize the treatment more. He proposed starting radiation immediately and, in light of how fast this thing was growing, we all concurred. After Gene's treatment, we met with the center social worker who told us about other services and gave us a tour. By the end of the day, whichever staff member was looking for us would call for "the family." I guess it was obvious that we were all in this together.

We finally arrived home emotionally and physically exhausted. I saw Gene cry for about the second time in the 38 years I have known him, as he expressed his anger at God for allowing this to happen. I did not really feel angry; more disappointed and disillusioned as I saw the God I had considered loving, kind, and just putting such a good man through this hard trial. The next months would test, stretch, and reform our faith many times and in many ways.

Today Rob, Juli's husband, came out to spend the day with Gene while Jill, Juli and I drove to Portland to pick up daughter Jaimi and her son Kevin at the airport. They were flying in from their home in Germany. On our way home, we stopped to do a little retail therapy, looking for a new recliner for Gene. He had been spending about 15 hours a day in the old recliner we bought at the PX in Germany (about 20 years ago!) and it sure was not that comfy anymore. In fact, when he sits down in it, the seat sinks nearly to the floor.

We looked at some Lazy Boys in one store, picked one we liked, then tried to dicker on the price. They weren't into that so we decided to look down the street before making a decision. We picked one out at the next store and asked the clerk for the "Saturday Special Price" on it. She laughed and asked what that would be. We named a number about $50 less than the ticket price and she agreed to it. Seconds later, an angry looking woman swept out of the adjacent office, grabbed the tags out of our clerk's hands and said, "You can't do that. Don't ever do that!" We were stunned that she would embarrass her employee and us in that way so turned and walked out of the store.

As we walked down the street marveling over the incident, Jill said, "I'm going back to say something to her." I went with her. We walked up to the angry woman and asked if she was the manager. She told us she owned the store. We told her we could not believe she would treat her employee and customers like that for $50. I said if I

8

were her employee, I would have walked out of the store and never come back and that's what we, the customers, were going to do. As we walked out, another employee caught my eye and gave us a "thumbs up."

We went back to the Lazy Boy store and told them we had found another chair but the owner was so rude to her employee that we walked out. The guy said, "Store X?" naming the store. Apparently her reputation preceded us. Anyway, we told the guy we wanted the chair but needed a swivel put on it. As he worked on the chair, Jill called home to give Rob an ETA. She asked me if I wanted Rob to feed the horses. The furniture guy asked about the horses, and before you know it, we had arranged to trade a horse for the chair. He got a heckuva deal on the horse, but I need to get rid of about 10 of them considering the big change our lives are making, so it was a good deal for me too. But the best part was the great laughs we get every time we think about trading a horse for a chair. We told the guy he should rename the pony Lazy Boy and we would call the chair Midy after the horse.

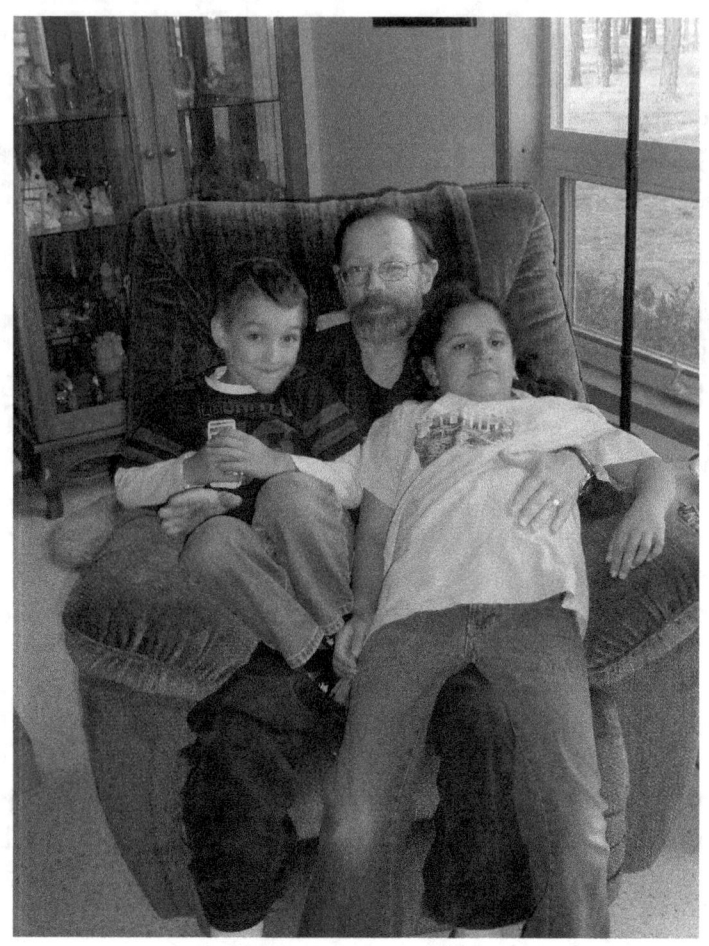
Papa Gene's chair is the place to be!

SUNDAY, OCTOBER 29, 2006 10:58 AM

Today was a family day. We had planned to take the kids to a special event at Maryhill Museum but we were all so wiped out we decided we just needed a quiet day at home together. Papa Gene helped each of the kids choose a pumpkin from the garden and we had a fine time carving them up into

10

all sorts of crazy jack-a-lanterns. Rob (our own personal Chef Ramsey) fixed a turkey dinner. Gene was able to eat a little of it.

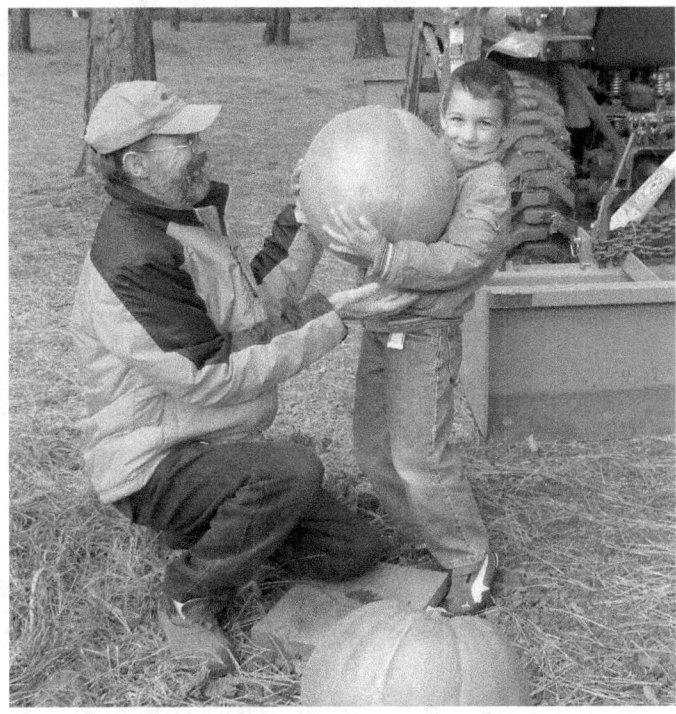

Gene helps Kevin with his choice.

TUESDAY, OCTOBER 31, 2006 11:08 AM

Today was Gene's third radiation treatment. He is scheduled for every day probably for 6 weeks, but this will be more formally set when Dr. Steltzer has the results of a treatment planning CT and a PET scan, which we made appointments for this week.

We also met for the first time with Dr. Taylor, who is the chemo doctor. He was not happy with the ambiguity of the pathology report. The report says the mass is "probably non-small cell lung

11

cancer" but this indefinite diagnosis is more based on what they ruled out than on a clear picture of what is really going on. This makes it tough for Dr. Taylor to plan treatment, so he scheduled Gene to have the biopsy re-done tomorrow in hopes of getting a better sample and a better diagnosis.

Gene has been really sick and unable to eat the last couple of days. We assume it is the pain medication, so Dr. Taylor wrote a prescription for a different one. Gene is so thin he really can't afford to lose any more weight. He has lost 3 pounds since Friday, so almost a pound a day.

FRIDAY, NOVEMBER 03, 2006
11:15 AM

It has been a hectic week. We drive every day to The Dalles for treatment and other appointments. Wednesday, we spent most of the day there to redo the biopsy. Gene is doing a little better on the new pain medication but still only eating things like soup and yogurt. I make him a shake every night with Ensure, ice creAM fruit and protein powder. He manages about 8 ounces of it.

Yesterday Jaimi took Gene over for his treatment and the treatment planning CT. I spent the day with Kevin and Ellie. It was a nice break, but maybe relaxed me too much because I had a bad night last night. I have been holding together pretty well, but finally came unglued. I decided to start this site as a distraction and outlet and spent until 3:00 am getting it set up and writing the preceding entries to get caught up to date.

12

Today was a horribly long day. Jaimi, Jill and I drove with Gene to The Dalles for his treatment, then on to Portland for the PET scan. We were all wiped out. When we got to Juli's to pick up the kids, she told us her co-teacher, Rachele, and Rachele's mom, Renee, had brought over a complete lasagna dinner for all of us. How nice not to have to worry with dinner after a long day. Thank you so much, ladies!

SATURDAY, NOVEMBER 04, 2006
11:22 AM

Today is Saturday so we didn't have to go anywhere! What a relief! Juli, Rob and kids came up and we all just hung out. Gene drug out a puzzle which they finished today. Kevin spent hours sitting on Gene's lap in the new recliner. He seems to need lots of Papa Gene time which, of course, breaks Gene's heart.

Gene felt a lot better today. Still tired and needing naps, but eating a little better. And I got him outside for a little walk during a sun break in what has been a very wet and rainy week. We fed apples to the horses and petted the babies. Great therapy!

Leslie (Gene's sister) called and we asked her bunches of questions. She has been a great support to us. She is a nurse so has lots of medical knowledge and also advice on nutrition, meds, etc.

Tomorrow, Jaimi and Kevin go home.

Sunday Juli and Jill took Jaimi and Kevin to the airport while Rob and kids hung out here with us. Kalle and Ellie stayed busy with Barbies while Dillon shot pool and built things with a new construction toy Jill brought home. Gene mostly slept and Rob labored away in the kitchen on some world class Jambalaya.

Monday was a rough day. We talked to Dr. Steltzer about the PET scan. A couple of spots showed up on the liver and one on the spine. I was pretty devastated that the cancer has spread but Gene, with his usual optimism, said, "What's a little spot on the liver and spine. Chemo will take care of that."

He had his first acupuncture treatment, too. We are hoping it will help with the nausea and pain. The acupuncturist showed me some pressure points to work on at home, and he will go in for treatment twice a week.

Today we met with Dr. Taylor (chemo) again. He is expecting the new biopsy report by the end of the week, but is pretty much on hold until then.

The center offers free massage for patients and caregivers, so today during a long wait between appointments, I opted for a massage while Gene took a nap in the meditation room. Robin, the massage therapist, wondered where the girls were today. We have shown up en masse pretty much everyday so that all the staff just refers to us as "The Family". Jill says it makes her feel Italian.

14

Thanks to Esther and Donna for bringing us dinner the past two days! Esther, one of our church friends, has offered to coordinate meal deliveries on treatment days. It is so nice to have one less thing to deal with and the food is great too!

I have been printing out the email messages and Guestbook entries for Gene to read. He (and we all) appreciate so much all the love and support you are all pouring out to us. Gene said he wished he felt well enough to answer all these messages and asked if I was keeping up with them. Sorry if I'm not, but please know how much we appreciate you all.

From the Guest book

WEDNESDAY, NOVEMBER 08, 2006

There once was this dude named Gene.

Who I called the Lean Mean Machine.

He was forced into a fight,

So with all of his might,

He showed us what courage does mean.

You've always been an inspiration Geno. Now you're just going to add to that legacy

Your buddy Big Al.

Vancouver, WA

THURSDAY, NOVEMBER 09, 2006

Conversation between Drill Sergeant and new recruit to Gene's Army:

"When He says you are a DORK, you are going to like it. DO YOU HEAR ME?

YES, Drill Sergeant!!

"When HE says you are FULL OF CRAP, you are going to like it. DO YOU HEAR ME?

YES, Drill Sergeant!!

"When HE calls you a DORK and says you are FULL OF CRAP, that means you are his FRIEND. DO YOU HEAR ME?

YES, Drill Sergeant!!

Big Al

THURSDAY, NOVEMBER 09, 2006
1:32 PM

Today we had good news. But first:

It's been a tough couple of days after the news on Monday. Gene has not felt at all well, still having a lot of trouble keeping food down. He is down to 135 pounds. The girls and I have been so anxious. Jaimi has booked a flight to come back next week and my dad is poised to come up for a visit. In the meantime, we have been praying that this is a germ cell tumor because Dr. Steltzer said that would be a more treatable option. I told Gene on Monday that the good thing about getting the bad news about the mets (metastases) was that anything coming after that could only be good news comparably.

Well, guess what! Today when we showed up for the daily radiation treatment, Linda, Dr. S's nurse, said, "both of you come back here. We have good news!" Yeehaw! Dr. S then explained that one of the blood tests on Monday had shown the marker for germ cell tumor to be very high. So without waiting further on the super slow biopsy path, he and Dr. T agreed to attack the cancer on

16

the marker evidence. So Dr. S sent us straight up to Dr. T who immediately started Gene on a chemo regimen. Germ cell tumors are very responsive to chemo so this is great news. However, one of the best drugs for this treatment can be hard on the lungs, so they agreed to stop the radiation immediately so as not to have that also blasting the tumor in the lungs. Gene has the drugs dripping into him as I write this and we are so happy that it now looks like we are dealing with a cancer with a possible cure and not just "buying time" which is what we were told Monday after the mets were found.

To add to the story, on Monday after the bad news, I was reading from my current good read by Nicholas Sparks, "Three Weeks with my Brother." I ran across a Bible verse I have seen and even quoted many times, but with a little different end to it than I have seen before. It went like this: "God keeps his Promise, and he will not allow you to be tested beyond your power to remain firm, at the same time, you are put to the test, he will give you the strength to endure it, and to provide you with a way out." I have taken issue with this passage a number of times in recent years when I have felt tested beyond my ability to endure with issues with our "Six Pack" of adopted kids. And the past few weeks, I really have taken issue with it, so when I read the part I do not remember reading before, "provide you with a way out." I asked God where the heck the way out was. Today I feel reaffirmed that he is still looking out for us in spite of our anger and hurt about "too much testing". Maybe we do have a way out!

Of course, chemo will not be a picnic, particularly with Gene already so thin, but knowing there is a bright spot in the future will sure help get through it. So do all of you! Gene laughed over some of the guest book messages, yesterday (and Mick, I can't believe he told you that I locked him out that night![1]) and they do give him strength in knowing everyone is behind him. So once again, thank you all!

FRIDAY, NOVEMBER 10, 2006
8:37 PM

Boy I am learning a lot more than I ever wanted to know. Gene is receiving three chemo drugs. Each one of those has nasty side effects, so he receives another six to nine drugs to combat the side effects. When they call in our prescriptions now, they just say "another one for Gene". Oh the joys of living in a small town!

Gene did so great yesterday. He was chipper all day and hardly slept at all. Then we got home and he was bustling around till I roped him and drug him to bed about 11. One of the drugs they give him for nausea is a steroid and it is making him feel great. We are calling it the Superman drug. Today was harder though. He got the hiccups this morning and they lasted all day. The nurse told us that some patients have them for days. Yikes! He was a lot more tired today and the chemo takes

---

[1]Mick and Gene first worked together on the Umpqua National Forest in Roseburg when Juli and Jaimi were tiny. I think Mick was the one who presented us with a Goddess of Fertility—I guess 2 kids seemed quite a lot to a guy whose only child at the time was a Porsche. Mick wrote in the guestbook a story of a performance evaluation that took place at a local bar, way into the night, resulting in a mad wife and a locked door.

18

forever. We left home at 7:15 am for the drive to the Dalles and got back here again at 6:30 pm. I am wiped out and I am healthy! I'm not sure how the patients manage it. I don't know what more the center could do to make it as easy as possible. It is a beautiful facility with lots of services, including a spa, exercise room, and meditation room (which we have used for naps--oh well, we meditate in our sleep). The chemo room has big windows with views of the gorge, they bring around juice, snacks and lunch, have little portable DVD players and a good selection of movies, comfy recliners, warm blankies and terrific staff. But still, what a long day! We get the weekend off though then back M,T,W for more drugs. He will be on a regimen of five days chemo, then 2 weeks rest. We are not sure how many cycles it will take but we are in it till he's well.

Juli and her friend Paula came and cleaned our house today. Paula even cleaned out the refrigerators. Now that's scary! I hope she doesn't catch some awful disease from stuff we had growing in there. And Juli taped "inspirational messages" all over the house: "Go Germy Gene, fight this thing!" "Go Go Go, drink H2O", "food is your friend" and on the underside of the toilet seat: "Now get back in there and EAT." Thanks ladies! I don't know how: a) people with jobs can deal with this--if either one of us had a real job we would be hosed and b) how we would do it still without the girls here. We normally leave home at 8:00 to take Kalle, Dori and Breanna to school, then pick them back up again at 3:00 (2:00 on Wed). Looks like we will be missing both ends of the transportation during chemo days, so Jill takes them in the morning (makes her about 45 minutes late to work) and Juli picks them up in the afternoon and keeps them till we get home. Of course, change in routine is really tough on Kalle, so that is an extra challenge, but so far she has done really well with it all. Jaimi is coming back for another week on the 16th, so she will be here for Gene's "off chemo" phase. Maybe he will be feeling better for this visit! He was pretty wasted last week when she was here; now we are realizing it was largely due to dehydration because he is feeling and eating much better now with all the fluids they are pumping into him along with the chemo.

So that is the life we are living now as we fight this awful beast. I realize that I have been fortunate not to have anyone really close to me going through such a serious illness before. I have a lot to learn about being there for Gene; I am afraid I hover too much and then leave him alone at the wrong time to compensate. Oh well, we are all learning.

The prayers are working; please keep them flying!

SUNDAY, NOVEMBER 12, 2006
4:44 PM

Happy "He Still Has Hair" Day!! Juli and Rob decided our weekly Sunday family gathering should be themed around commemorating Dad's hair while he still has some!! And they have put on such an event that Christmas will pale in comparison. After Juli's major Portland shopping excursion yesterday, they arrived with presents for the whole family, games and books and food for the "patient" and a roast that is supposed to look like hair when it is done cooking. Unfortunately, the guest of honor

20

has lost some steam and is sleeping through the big fiesta, and we have had to postpone the "mane" event, a new game befitting of our dad, titled "Fact or Crap". We decided the game would be best turned into a drinking game, tequila shots for us, water for the patient who is 32 ounces behind his daily intake. (Juli said it was a BYOW day, and brought a whole case of bottled water that has yet to be cracked open!) So we anxiously await his return to consciousness and to our party. In the meantime, we sit and wait, "combing" through catalogs, "brushing" up on our crosswords, and "highlighting" some crappy facts that we think will "shed'" some light on the need for dad to eat and drink more voraciously (Juli says, "you mean, at all?"), our biggest challenge.

Juli thinks she must be the one who puts her dad to sleep, because yesterday he had a pretty energetic day. First thing in the morning, our neighbor, Chuck, showed up looking for work. Gene went out and got him lined up to drag the road with the tractor. Thanks Chuck, your 14 passes got most of the potholes out of there!! Then, Gene was so happy to be outside, he spent about an hour working in the garden and brushing beets for winter storage.

Well, time to go check on the roast and on the dad.

Fact or Crap: Tomorrow, Dad will spend 2.5 hours in the car, 7 hours with 10 different drugs (aka poison) dripping into his vein, approx 120 minutes listening to us say drink some water, and still manage to nag mom about whether she has given Kalle her spelling words.

21

You got it: FACT (that is, "bald" truth!)....and yes, it is a lot of CRAP, too!!

Judi, Juli, and Jill

P.S. Thanks, Kip, for the bottle of wine!! It has been a great aid in writing this hair-raising entry!!

MONDAY, NOVEMBER 13, 2006
7:07 PM

Well our FACT for today ended up being CRAP.

Dad missed his Chemo treatment because he had to go for an ambulance ride to a hospital in Portland!!!

He woke up at about four in the morning feeling really horrible, and mom said looked worse than that, and after a few excruciating hours they took off for The Dalles ER. There the doctors were afraid that he was having a heart attack, or a ruptured artery, caused by the radiation-due to the proximity of the tumor to his heart. SCARY!!!! So dad took off in the ambulance, mom in the suburban and the rest of us ran around Goldendale, like chickens with our heads cut off, getting out of work, hunting down husbands, picking up kids and rounding up help for the animals. By the time dad came out of the cath lab, and mom called with better-than-worse news, I was ready to have a nervous breakdown! Thankfully (I guess) the diagnosis is fluid around the heart. I'm sure my mom will elaborate with the correct terminology later. They will both stay there for the night and are planning on coming home tomorrow.

22

My mom said my dad came out of the cath lab feeling pretty good and even ate a huge dinner, I think that guy just needs a permanent IV bag attached to him! Lucky for Dad, Prison Break is on tonight (TV), not so lucky, so is the Bachelor. Not too sure who is going to win that one in the ICU! I don't know what this setback does to continuing treatment, I guess we'll just have to wait and see. Rob decided we should all learn a little lesson from today: that we need to have some kind of emergency plan ready for action. The problem is can you really ever prepare for anything like this??? There was also a positive note, since mom and dad were MIA, my family (along with Jill, Kalle, Dori & Breanna,) had a wonderful dinner prepared by friends Esther and Kim. And wouldn't you know, it was spaghetti! (MY favorite!) Thanks ladies, the pumpkin cake was amazing, and we even saved some for mom & dad!

All kidding aside, this battle is really hard...and heartbreaking...and we are so thankful for all of you that are praying and caring for my dad and us!

Hoping for a better day tomorrow!

Juli

TUESDAY, NOVEMBER 14, 2006
9:48 PM

We're B-A-A-A-C-K.

Yup, this is Judi again, broadcasting from the ark. That Hair Celebration really kicked off a couple of hair raising days. I don't think we will try that again! I have never seen anyone in that much

23

pain. I made it to The Dalles in about 45 minutes. I usually allow a little over an hour for the trip from the ranch to the hospital. But I was pretty sure he was gonna kick the bucket before I got there so I did some hair raising driving. When we got to the ER, they did an EKG and determined that he was having a heart attack, gave him 4 baby aspirin, pumped him full of nitro and thrombolytics and put him in an ambulance for Portland. The good news is that it was actually just pericarditis (not that that made it any less painful). It is weird that the EKG looked for all the world like an MI and in fact, the EKG machine analysis labeled it as acute infarct. But the angiogram showed no damage or blockages and the ultrasound also was normal, so he is taking Motrin for pain and inflammation. It's kind of funny that with all the fancy drugs they gave him in the ER, probably the baby aspirin was the only one that helped any! In retrospect, I am convinced this has been his pain all along, not the tumor, and that it was our clue to get him examined to find the cancer. Okay, God, we get it, now enough with the chest pain!

Two other bad things (besides a lot of pain, hair raising trip to The Dalles and then Portland, and a long couple of days): One, we missed two days of chemo so are really off schedule and two, our friends Marilyn and Earl showed up at Celilo to keep us company on Monday and we never showed! Bummer!

As for the chemo, we stopped to talk to Dr. Taylor on the way home from Portland and he is planning on a double dose tomorrow, then go on break as planned for the rest of this week and next, starting in with the full five days the following week.

So tomorrow will be a very long day (what? again?!?) but then hopefully some quiet time. Jaimi will be home Thursday night, so some good family time this weekend, hoping Gene will not be puking his guts out the whole time. . .

I do not know how we would do this without the girls and all our friends. Jill got everyone (horses, dogs, cat, birds, kids) taken care of this morning, then Juli picked kids up after school. This is getting pretty routine for her since we are often not home in time to get them. She is even managing to get Kalle's homework done! Whew. When we got home, we stopped at Juli's to get the kids and Kimmy, our pastor, was there delivering dinner. Spanikopita tonight. It was awesome. Jill says she will actually miss this part, but I reminded her that we are probably gaining a pound for every one Gene loses. Seriously though, when Esther offered to arrange meals for us, I felt like that would be such an imposition on people and we really are able bodied and should be able to do this ourselves. But what a blessing to come home and have great food with no thought and no work! So it is appreciated more than I could ever have imagined. And we also found a beautiful cherry pie sitting on the cupboard when we got home. My friend Marilyn makes the best cherry pie in the world and this looked (and tasted!) like hers, but actually another friend, Connie, dropped this one off at Juli's. I did not know two people could make pie like this! All right: let's go for a cook off.

Gene was wiped out today but Dr. Taylor gave him some anti-nausea meds, including the Superman drug, and by supper time, he actually ate some real food and got to acting like his dorky

25

obnoxious self. He even ate cherry pie and ice cream with John and Doug who were our straw delivery angels tonight. Thanks guys!

It is probably becoming obvious that I am half delirious. I am so tired! This journal has become a real outlet for all of us. Sometimes we get a little silly and it feels good. The truth is, many of our moments and hours are filled with fear and exhaustion

Oh, but another piece of fun news: Our favorite Dr, who was in the ER on one of our pain visits and you have read about tracking us down a number of times, showed up in The Dalles ER yesterday while we were there. He happened to be in town (doing a neurological study day, I think he said) and heard we were there and just popped over to check on us. Is he incredible!

Does anyone notice that we have a lot of angels in our lives?

WEDNESDAY, NOVEMBER 15, 2006
9:22 PM

I am brilliant!

Marilyn took the bait and delivered a peach pie today! Let the games begin!

Even better, Marilyn and Earl gave us another chance after our no show at the clinic on Monday and came by again today. Marilyn took me out to lunch and Earl sat and visited with Gene. We all had a great time! Thanks so much, dear friends! If you don't know about Marilyn and Earl, we first met them in Roseburg in 1972 when we backed over the top of their VW with our truck. And now she bakes us pies. Go figure!

Anyway, their visit sure helped get through a very long day. We were at the clinic from 9:00 till 6:15 or so. Yows! But no more chemo till after Thanksgiving. YEEHAW. Hopefully Gene will get over the pukes in time for Thanksgiving dinner.

Speaking of the pukes, we came to the conclusion that the "never sick a day in his life" guy's stomach just refuses to deal with pills. Every time he has to take his medicine he gets sick. So we spent part of today getting some of the pills re-prescribed in other forms (egs: he is now taking big gobs of liquid children's ibuprofen instead of pills. . . BTW, did I mention we got him clear off of morphine after figuring out the pain was pericarditis and NOT the giant tumor!?!?). And Kurt, our super nurse, gave him lessons in pill taking strategies for the ones that have to be in pill form. Who knew pill taking was such an art? Meanwhile, poor Gene is down to 128 pounds and dehydrates pretty fast so we are gonna get set up to give him IV fluids at home till we get the nausea thing under control.

We had meal deliveries from Diane and Dawn today, so have one saved for tomorrow! Rebecca came over to feed the horses since we knew none of us would be home till after dark. Thank you, all!

From the Guest book

TUESDAY, NOVEMBER 15, 2006

(Theme to Gilligan's Island)
Just sit right back and hear a tale,
A tale of a family.
That started from a ranch out west
Oh so fatefully.
The Dad was a might family man
The Mother brave and strong
The Children all set sail that day
To cure what just went wrong, To cure what just went wrong.
The battle started getting rough
The Dad was being tossed.
If not for the courage of the family
The Dad might be lost, The Dad might be lost.
They placed their faith in God above,
Relied on all their Friends.
They laughed and cried and really tried
To get Dad on the mend.
The chemo started taking hold
The tumor shrunk and shrunk
The Family all rejoiced with Hope,
The Dad couldn't wait to get drunk
The Friends, The Church, The Hospital
They were all on their side
They read the journal every day
They helped to turn the tide.
Then one day the X-ray cleared
The tumor wasn't there.

The Dad was back to his dorky self
He was so skinny he had nothing to wear.
So he drank that long awaited beer
He ate what food was brought
The Family was in such good cheer
The Dad was back to being a Snot.
So that my friends was a tale of Hope,
For all of you to see.
This miracle was brought to you
By the Cyrus Family!
Big Al

THURSDAY, NOVEMBER 16, 2006
6:22 PM

I got the day off today! Well, most of it anyway. Juli took Gene to The Dalles today for his daily drink of saline and acupuncture and I stayed home and got some of the neglected things (like changing the sheets, laundry, etc.) done. Then my friend Dawn came over and we had a great visit. I love to go with Gene and be with him for his treatment, but it was honestly a relief to not be there for a little while. It does get hard looking at his scrawny body and watching him feel bad but knowing of nothing to do to make him feel better. And I'm sure it was nice for him to have Juli there instead for a change. Fresh energy!

A lot of people have been asking about this weird form of cancer that Gene has, so I thought I would share some of the information we have gathered. Here are some interesting tidbits:

29

Germ cell tumors usually form in the gonads. Many researchers believe that extra-gonadal (not in the gonads) are related to developmental problems that occur before birth. In the growing embryo, germ cells typically move from a site near the middle of the body to their permanent home in the ovaries or testes. Sometimes, however there is a problem, and the germ cells never reach their final destination. Instead, they settle in the mid-chest area between the lungs, in the lower back, or in the middle of the brain. Sometimes these misplaced cells develop into tumors. Only 1 to 4% of germ cell tumors are extra-gonadal and about 40% of those tumors are cancerous. In fact, only one new case of cancerous non-gonadal germ cell tumor is diagnosed each year for every 2 million to 3 million people in the US. So you see that Gene really won the lottery here.

Prognosis: Long term survival is 75 – 80% after chemotherapy. Hence our excitement that the cancer was re-diagnosed as germ cell instead on non-small cell lung cancer with mets!

Gene called Al today to tell him that 2 of his women laughed and 1 cried when they read the Gilligan song. All of us are impressed with his creativity and diligence! I think we will all sing it at Gene's 60th birthday party (only 2 years away!). Maybe we can get Esther's husband, Doug, to record it along with the Dancing Mountain song he wrote for our retirement/Jill moving to Goldendale party.

Gene ate 2 pieces of pizza tonight (Thanks, Kip!) Go figure: we keep trying to think up nice bland, easy to eat things for him and then he gobbles up taco pizza. That's what I get for thinkin'!

Jill is in Portland now picking up Jaimi. They should be home about 10:00. Can't wait. And I am already wondering what Rob will cook for dinner Sunday. Jill saw Dr. Sherpa today and he said he was coming out to visit Sunday so maybe he will get in on some of Rob's great food.

MONDAY, NOVEMBER 20, 2006
12:59 AM

Well, RB complained about no updates for a few days so guess I'd better get on the stick. No news pretty much means things are holding steady. Gene is eating a little bit better so that is a move in the right direction. No chemo this week so hopefully he will continue to feel more like eating.

We had a lazy stay at home weekend. I never even got dressed yesterday. I can't believe it! I hoped to get to church today but by the time I got Gene situated (it takes a long time in the morning to get his medicine down one pill at a time without causing trouble) and Kalle moving, it was too late. But we had a nice day. Jaimi worked a puzzle, I did crosswords, then we all watched a movie with the kids. Rob outdid himself with my favorite meal yet-- sort of an Indian chicken dish on rice and Juli's famous carrots (yes, on occasion Juli DOES cook). Dr. Sherpa got here in time to join the dinner crowd so that was cool.

Gene is really sick of being sick. He is very low energy and also cold all the time (a combination of no body fat and dehydration). He wanted to drive up to the property this weekend to check it out but luckily we didn't make it. I was afraid it would be

31

depressing because I really dropped the ball on the work up there and most likely we would have gotten stuck in the mud. Jaimi is driving him to Celilo tomorrow for hydration and I am going to school with Kalle to be her moral support while she presents her science "project". She practiced on all of us this weekend but is still very nervous about talking in front of the whole class. Tuesday is a big day: CT scan and he gets a PICC line put in. Then we will be able to give him fluids at home, which will save us a lot of driving.

TUESDAY, NOVEMBER 21, 2006
9:53 PM

Whew. Another long day. It started out bad cuz Gene had to drink two big bottles of "Berry Smoothie" (Barium Sulphate contrast for the CT scan). He got most of the first one down but about the time we hit the bottom of the grade going to The Dalles it came back up. They did the CT anyway and then we went over to Celilo for his daily two bags of liquids. He weighed in at a mighty 125.6 pounds today :-(Hopefully this is the bottom for this round because the rest of the day he has eaten pretty well and no more puke buckets. That lovely breakfast smoothie was just too much!

We never caught up with Dr. Taylor today (I have the feeling he was avoiding us. I think maybe Jaimi and I together are a little overbearing) so do not know how the scan turned out. Jaimi is in charge of cornering him tomorrow as I have school duty. If nothing else, we actually have an appointment on Monday but that is a bit long to wait for any news. If there is any news. . .

Juli picked kids up again today because we didn't get home till about 4:00. Then it was time to feed horses, humans, etc. and get kids off to bed. Next week Juli will be the main mama all week since we will be back on the long chemo days.

We got some more neat messages on the guest book today! Fun how all the old friends and relatives are checking in. We also got this great email from Cabuya school (the school in Panama that we visited in 2005 with gifts from Kalle's school, uniforms bought by the Goldendale Kiwanis, and lots of other gifts and party things). Anyway, it says (roughly translated): "Mr. Gene Cyrus: Best regards to you and we are praying to God for your quick recovery. In the name of members of the school, teachers, students, and the Family of the Students Club of Cabuya we are praying for your health and hope you are well soon. Regards for your wife and your dear daughter who we always remember for the lovely gesture you made to our Community." We received a scan of this letter from our friend Mayra who has an employee from Cabuya. Apparently he took news of Gene's illness home with him and the school responded. Isn't it amazing how you can make little connections like this in your life and have them come back in such heartfelt ways? And we also got the guestbook message from Ernesto, another friend in Panama, about putting Gene's name in his international prayer chain. I have this vision of all these prayers wafting up to heaven from all around the world. What a blessing to feel surrounded by such love!

Tomorrow I am doing kid pickup and drop off cuz school is out at noon and I anyway have a date with Rob to go to Ellie's preschool "feast". Since Juli is the teacher, she can't actually be a guest so Rob and I are the family reps. Then I'm gonna get the pre stuff done for Thanksgiving dinner since the plan is for Jill to stay home with Gene tomorrow night while I take Jaimi to Portland and stay over to see her off early Thursday morning. I will then come home early to get dinner finished. Gene's a little nervous about me being gone (me too, but also looking forward to a night out with Jaimi and maybe Juli will go too). Jaimi will be flying home to Germany on Thanksgiving Day so will miss the big feast, but she and Kevin will be back on Dec. 11, so we will just look forward to that!

From the amount of food Gene put away today, I am thinking the plan for him to be ready for Thanksgiving dinner is working out! I think he will have to eat the whole turkey to get built up for next weeks ordeal!

Happy Thanksgiving everyone! Please know that each of you will be on our "thanks" list especially this day.

FRIDAY, NOVEMBER 24, 2006
10:02 AM

Fact or Crap: Gene ate a huge Thanksgiving dinner and didn't even puke it up.

Wednesday was a rough day. When Gene and Jaimi got home from Celilo he was feeling pretty puny so we decided Jill and Juli should take Jaimi to the airport and I would stay home. Good thing. It was a rough evening.

Then he woke up Thursday morning feeling pretty good. Ate breakfast then started in on turkey parts. By noon he had finished off the gizzard, heart and neck (now THAT would make ME sick!) At 2:00 he joined the gang at the dinner table and polished off a plate of turkey (the wing, not his usual drumstick: that was just TOO daunting), dressing, sweet potatoes, green bean casserole, cranberries and pickled beets. Then he rested for about 45 minutes and did it again! We could not believe it. I was a little worried about Plate Two but all was well! Later he ate a sliver of each kind of pie (Rob's pumpkin and pecan and my marionberry) and ice cream. Whew! and Yeehaw! Jill took a picture of him with the dinner but I can't find it on her camera. When we find it, I will put it in the photo section. It was truly a memorable occasion!

He is feeling good this morning, too. I guess he finally got over the last round of chemo. Just in time to fatten him up a little before next week. Dr. Sherpa left standing orders at the hospital so we could take him in for fluids this weekend but so far it does not look like we will have to do that. A little break! Four days at home would be just fine with me.

SATURDAY, NOVEMBER 25, 2006
5:11 PM

HI GUYS!

Yes, it's really me. [Gene speaking]. After a horrendously crappy week and a half, I am finally starting to feel somewhat human again. So I wanted to take this opportunity to personally reply

35

to all of you that have done so much to make me feel better. Judi prints out the messages every day for me to read and they truly make my day! You make me chuckle, you remind of great memories, you overwhelm me with your thoughts and prayers, you make me realize how truly full my life has been. I wish I could reply to each of you individually but please know how much I treasure each one of your messages. It makes me humble (hard to believe, hey?) to hear from so many friends and loved ones from all over the world.

Your messages give me peace and comfort at the moment while helping to build my strength for the next round in this little skirmish. Also, know how much Judi, Juli, Jaimi and Jill appreciate reading them. You buoy their spirits as well and they are so strong and supportive in helping me through this.

Got another round of chemo coming up starting Monday (Ugh!) so the next round begins. In the meantime, I'll try to add some meat to my poor puny bones.

Thanks again for being there and for being such an important part of my life. What a support group! Love you guys a bunch. Will write again soon.

And remember, nobody is totally worthless; they can always be used as a bad example. [The editor preferred to axe this remark but in the interest of journalistic integrity, refrained.]

Gene

Well, day one of round two went amazingly well! Gene felt pretty good all day and went home and thoroughly enjoyed a meatloaf dinner delivered by Buzz and Sue. He even ate apple crisp and ice cream for dessert! He weighed in at 130 pounds this morning! Yeehaw!

Sunday was our family day. Rob got called out to work so Juli and kids rode home with me after church but Rob showed up in time to cook the turkey soup and sloppy joes (I know, strange menus but the sloppy joes were Gene's request. He did eat them but returned them later :-(However, he has not sent anything back since then!

The really great part about Sunday was that Gene bundled up and pulled the kids on sleds behind the tractor! They all had fun (especially Gene). Juli and I worked on thank you cards (her mom-in-law, sis-in-law and friend Tracy have been keeping us supplied but we thought we should get some done too). And since there was about 6 inches of snow on the ground, we all enjoyed hanging out around the fire.

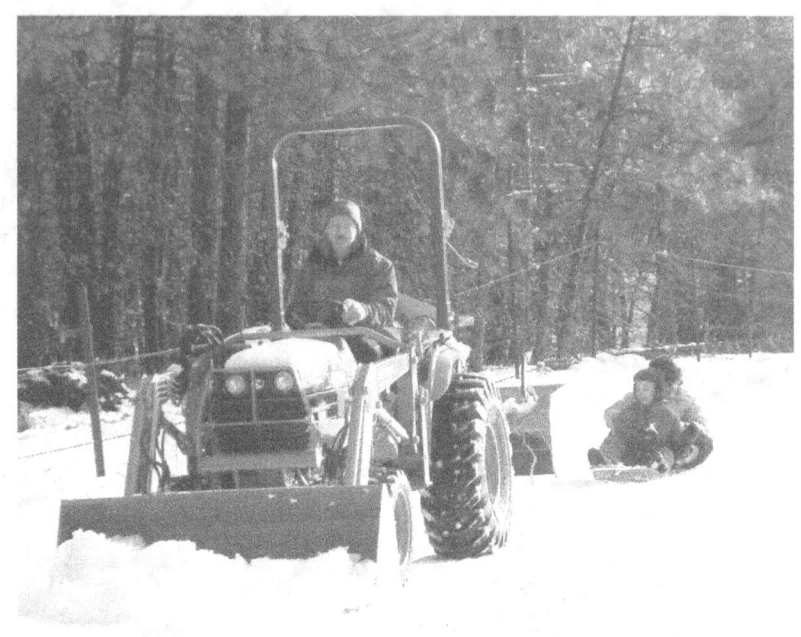

Yesterday went by pretty fast thanks to visits from Dr. Sherpa and Sandi, Kalle and Dillon's kindergarden teacher, a cancer survivor herself. Now we're back at Celilo for Day 2 as I type this. My plan for the day is to work for awhile (I was lucky enough to get a little job from Heartstream), then go in the spa, then do a little shopping (Kalle needs some gloves!) Gene is getting a foot massage then has some crosswords waiting for him. It'll be another long day but we are kind of getting used to it.

Our big hope for this week is that Gene keeps feeling good through tomorrow so we can go to the Trail Band concert. It has become something of a tradition to go with our friends Doug and Esther. Gene missed out last year cuz he was in Atlanta so he'll be bummed if he misses it again!

WEDNESDAY, NOVEMBER 29, 2006
8:56 PM

Day 3 of chemo cycle 2 and Gene is still eating and feeling good! Wow! Of course "good" is a little relative; he is worn out but believe it or not, hasn't puked since Sunday! I guess he LIKES getting his veins pumped full of poison!

Kalle was badly in need of a "normal" day, so Jill drove Gene to Celilo today and I did the kid runs so I could drop off and pick up Kalle and help her with homework like a normal day. She was very cuddly and sweet so think she needed some mommy time (and of course it fills me up too!)

Since I was home and doing the running, I had a more first hand experience on the whole meal thing. Our friend Esther has taken on the task of making sure we have meals on the LONG chemo days. Since on those days, Juli picks up all the kids (hers and ours), the way the meals work is that Esther, who works at the school, has the preparers drop the food off there, then transfers it to Juli. Then when we pick up the kids, we also pick up dinner. It's all very easy on our end and I shamefully admit I had not really thought about how complicated it really was until today when I was a more active participant and the meal did not have to change hands three times. It makes me even more grateful for the "easy" evenings when we breeze in after dark, pick kids and food up from Juli's where she has already dealt with homework, run on home, stick ready-to-eat food in the oven or microwave to warm, then run out to feed horses in the dark and come back in to an oh-so-easy hot

39

meal. And it is fun to eat someone else's cooking, too! Last night we had sausage casserole prepared by Kalle's teachers (along with big, juicy seedless grapes; I think Esther let out the word that grapes are one thing Gene seems to eat no matter how sick he is. The price of grapes will probably skyrocket in Goldendale due to the current high demand.) and tonight we had a chicken and stuffing dish with tropical fruit salad from Betty. And I have to confess that I got into the apple spice cake early while Kalle and I did homework.

Oh and I got to feed the horses in the daylight tonight before Jill and Gene got home. So they came home to chores all done, house pretty clean, fire blazing in the stove (we usually get home to a cold house :-(, and dinner already warm. Not bad for a chemo day.

We did, however, pass on the Trail Band concert. We are bummed, but Gene just felt too tired to add more to the end of the day. He was pleased to give the tickets to one of the nurses at Celilo who was excited to have them because the concert has been the talk of the center all week.

Tomorrow we are back to our regular schedule so here's hoping Kalle can get through two more long days without much mom and dad time. Then we get two weeks of more normal lives before Round Three!

Hello all - this is Jaimi. I've been an active journal reader / treatment chauffeur / humour booster / and fellow commiserator over the past few weeks. Kevin and I have been lucky enough to really maximize being with our family over these couple of months running up to the end of the year, and it is really important to us both. I thought maybe I would share how much of an impression being with "Papa Gene" made on Kevin. We spent a week over there, where Kevin spent hours per day on Papa Gene's lap in the recliner. When we got home again we were having a little chat while going to bed and talked about the movie Aladdin (which he had watched while we were there). I asked Kevin what he would wish for if he, like Aladdin, was granted 3 wishes. Here is what he said:

tapping chin and thinking... "my first wish would be..(finger in the air like a light bulb came on)...that Papa Gene gets well! And my second wish would be...that Papa Gene can wrestle with me again! And after that...hmmm (tapping his head this time)... I KNOW! that we could live forever with Baba and Papa Gene together!"

So we will be happy to get back there again in a couple weeks. In the meantime, I would like to also extend my thanks to everyone who is helping out so much - in actions, in words, and in prayers. It is hard to be far away and not able to contribute all the time, but I can rest easier knowing there are so many wonderful friends and family members out there, pulling together to help my parents and sisters get through each day. THANKS!

SATURDAY, DECEMBER 02, 2006
5:06 PM

Well, it was nice while it lasted, but the chemo finally caught up with Gene on Thursday night and he is feeling real poorly again. It was a blessing that he got through four days of it feeling pretty well though and able to eat pretty normally. The last day was not much fun, but he actually got through this round much better than the first (thanks to no extra goodies like fake heart attacks and double doses of chemo) so we are hoping the sickness will pass faster too. At least we know it will pass and then we are halfway through the planned treatment!

His last great meal was chicken enchiladas from church friends Janet and Dave (and Dave made the enchiladas--he and Rob should open a restaurant). He did manage a little of Sandi's yummy stew Friday night but unfortunately it did not stay with him long. So after a tough night last night, we dropped into the hospital today for a couple bags of fluids. Not the most exciting way to spend a sunny Saturday but hey, kidneys are good to keep around.

Jill and I are cooking Thai food tomorrow to give Rob a break. If the weather stays cold, maybe we can manage to move a load or so of hay, too. Or maybe we will be back at the hospital getting fluids. The night will tell.

Oh yeah, the hair is definitely going. The back of Gene's head has rubbed off like a baby's. He looks kind of like a baby bird with messy little feathers over bald spots. Dillon put a good face on it though and tells everyone he thinks Papa will look even better bald.

Next week should be an easier week. Gene has an ultrasound on Monday to check for pericardial effusion as a follow-up to the fake heart attack and Tuesday we meet with Dr. Taylor. Other than that, it will just be whatever we need to do to keep him hydrated. They did get his PICC line put in Wednesday, so we need to get home health up here to train us to run the fluids ourselves. Jill is disgusted that we have to be trained cuz she runs IV's in dogs all the time :-) But anyway, once we can do that, it will save us a lot of running. So this week, we are praying for lots of rest (for all of us!) and overcoming the nausea from this round.

WEDNESDAY, DECEMBER 06, 2006
10:53 AM

Well, Gene is still feeling pretty lousy. However, we are trying something new. I kept telling the nurses here that his retching did not seem like normal nausea; it would come on suddenly without notice and then afterwards he could eat with no problem. I also noticed that he has become increasingly agitated. Can't get comfortable, can't sleep, legs are jumping all the time and even some shaking. So I told the doc all this yesterday and also that I thought maybe the retching was related to this behavior (like a nervous reaction) and not true nausea. He said, HMMM. the composine might be doing that. Well, compasine is what he takes for nausea so the sicker he got the more he took, and well, you can guess the rest. So

43

we have dropped the compazine (okay, I can't spell, which is it?) and he is taking benadryl to counteract what might be an allergic reaction to the compazine. At the very least, he slept better last night (knocked out by the benadryl, most likely) and he has not upchucked in 24 hours!

We are at the clinic now, getting his daily dose of fluids but we are looking forward to an exciting evening. Steve from NC, Bud and Mike from TN and Dale from ID are all blowing in this afternoon for a visit! We first met Dale in about 1972 in Roseburg, OR, then this whole gang worked together and became our family when we were in Germany (1985-1989), then Steve and Bud also were in Panama with us (1997-1999) AND then all these guys worked with SBA last year for the Katrina disaster recovery stint! So this should be a real morale boost for Gene even though he thinks he is too sick for company. I told him he doesn't have to put on a big show, Steve will tell jokes and they will all entertain each other and Gene can just relax and enjoy.

Oh yeah, back to the doctor's visit yesterday. Gene's blood chemistry looked good. He still has great oxygenation and blood pressure. So there is some payback for being healthy all his life if after two rounds of super chemo, his body is still holding strong in most respects! The next round of chemo will be the week before Christmas :-(and after that they will do another CT scan to see where we are. The plan is still for four rounds.

WEDNESDAY, DECEMBER 06, 2006
9:54 PM

Two entries in one day might be a bit much, but I just had to get on to post this picture of Gene and his buddies. What a great evening we had with these good friends! Thanks, guys, for making the trip out here to see Gene. You made our day! We love you guys.

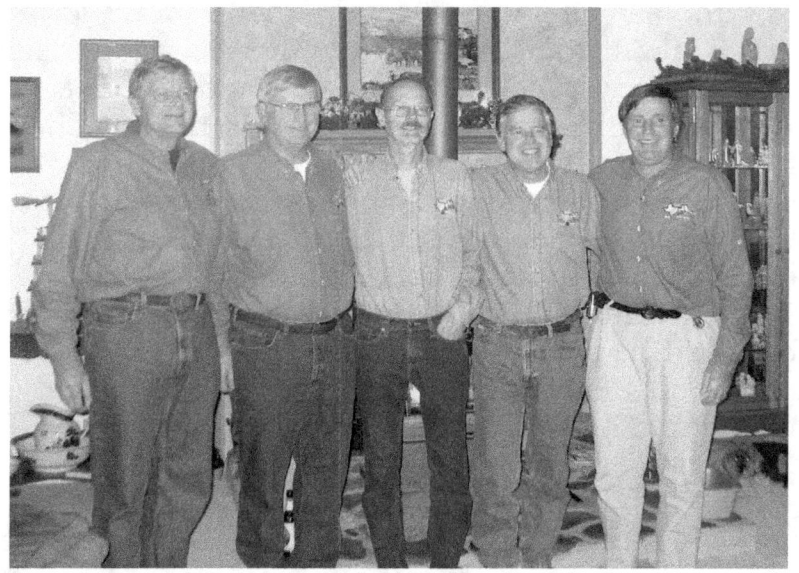

Bud, Steve, Gene, Mike and Dale

THURSDAY, DECEMBER 07, 2006
9:26 PM

It was another long day. It started out great and ended good, but the middle was long.

We met the "boys" at Sodbusters for breakfast and had some good laughs about Steve's

45

snoring (Bud drew the short stick and had Steve for
a roommate) and just enjoyed everyone's company.
We remembered a ski trip in Switzerland when
Steve, always early to retire, woke to all of us
standing around his bed watching him snore in
rhythm with the CD he had playing through his
headphones. Then we headed for Celilo and Gene's
daily hydration. By the time we got there, he was
feeling pretty puny and lay around in a fog all day.
The out-of-towners dropped by for a little while to
visit and say so-longs so that perked him up for a
little while. It was pretty funny; the receptionist led
all four of those big guys back to the treatment
room and our fun nurse Kurt started hurling chairs
at them, shouting "incoming" until there were
enough for all of them to sit down in our tiny room.
After they left, Gene pretty much passed out again
and Nina, the nurse practitioner spent the rest of
the day coming up with a new "feel better" regimen
for him. She says it is NOT okay that he is feeling
so crummy. So she called in Rx and I went
shopping. She also managed to get stuff
coordinated for us to do the fluid infusions at
home. We have been asking for this for several
weeks to save driving to The Dalles every day to sit
around there for hours but our insurance was not
real cooperative with the company in Goldendale
that does home health. So Nina finally arranged to
dispense the stuff from there. One of the nurses
had told us they could not do that but finally Nina
said she would just work it out, and a nurse is
coming out tomorrow with a pump, etc. Then we
will be good to go. So tomorrow we stay home!
Yeehaw! And no hospital trips for fluids this
weekend either.

So that rest we have been praying for may be coming soon!

My state Pony of the Americas club awards party is Sunday in Vancouver so was thinking about taking the kids but Jaimi is coming in Monday and I want to go pick her up so probably will stay home Sunday. I could probably make decisions better if my brain wasn't fried. I feel like I am wandering around in a fog. We'll see! Can't wait to see Jaimi and Kevin.

Oh yeah--and I mentioned that the day ended well too. We got home about 4:00 and I got the fire going and Gene and Kalle settled then went out to do my chores in the already almost dark. I had used up all the hay on the ground floor of the barn so was dreading climbing the ladder to the loft and throwing more down. But when I got to the barn, the hay bay on the ground was full! Our visitors had snuck back out here after breakfast and moved hay for me! Thanks guys!

SATURDAY, DECEMBER 09, 2006
5:28 PM

Yesterday was a hard day for me. I was looking forward to it because we did not have to go to Celilo (the home health nurses were coming to get us set up to do hydration at home) so I planned on taking a shower after I got home from taking the kids to school. Now, this is gross, but I had not taken a shower all week. Frankly, I don't have time! Previous weeks, I had been showering at Celilo in the spa while Gene was there anyway, but this week, he has felt so bad that I hated to leave him just to lounge in the spa and shower. So I didn't.

Yeah, gross. So you see why I was looking forward to a day at home.

It started out kind of nice because I didn't have to get Gene up and out of the house so he could relax in bed with his breakfast while I ran the kids in. But when I got home, there was a message on the machine from Kalle's school that she had head lice and I needed to call. Head lice have been going around all year and Kalle had them earlier. I have been combing her hair a couple of times a week with a lice removing comb and I actually bought some shampoo that is supposed to get them out, but when I read the directions, I decided I could not use it on her (it has all kinds of warnings on the label, one being that you must keep your eyes closed the whole ten minutes the stuff is on the hair, yeah, right. Kalle????) So I explained all this to the office staff and she told me she understood but that she had found something milder at KC pharmacy. I said, okay I would get that. But she said I had to come take Kalle home right now. So the whole school probably has head lice but because Kalle is in special ed (they also have combs and toothbrushes in their little boxes there that they use to learn personal hygiene—they comb their hair, brush teeth and wash hands when they come into class, which is cool but can't you just see them all using the wrong combs, ugh, and toothbrushes?), she gets checked and has to come home. I ranted a bit about they might as well just close the school down because even if I come and get her, she will still have lice tomorrow and will be back. . . But it is policy, so off I went to pick her up. I was so mad, frustrated, disappointed (no shower again???) that I bawled all the way into town. It is a 25 minute drive each way, so by now I am up to wasting two hours in the car and I will still have to go back in the afternoon to pick up Dori and Breanna. Anyway, I managed to get it together by the time I got to school and went in to get Kalle. They had sent her back to class (????) so I went to get her. She had her PE shoes on so I stood in the hall while she went in to change. While I was waiting, her teacher came out and asked how Gene was doing. Well, that was that and I started blubbering again. She gave me a big hug and I felt like a dork (but the hug was good). But I keep thinking that I am trying to help Gene get through cancer and I can't even get rid of head lice. . . After that, I decided I was not making another trip to town this day (not to mention that I did not know what time home health was coming and needed to be home for them) so I went to Dori and Breanna's school and said I needed to take them out. I did not offer any explanation but the principal took one look at my red face and swollen eyes and did not even ask (the cancer card. . .) I am a dork but you have all heard of the straw that broke the camel's back. Well, this camel is limping badly!

So came home, eventually home health showed up and about 7:00 that night I finally got a bath.

The good news is that the new anti vomit regimen seems to be working pretty well AND we now have home hydration. Zofran seems to be the only drug that really helps the nausea. It used to be $28 a pill, but just went generic so now we can get a whole bottle of it for $5! Gene has had a terrible sore throat the past couple of days though so still has felt miserable. He is a little better today so hopefully by tomorrow we will really be on the

49

upswing (just in time for Jaimi and Kevin to arrive Monday!)

Today Jill, Kalle and I went out with sleds and cross country skis to look for a Christmas tree. We tried to harness Luna (Jill's dog) to the sled but she managed to jump out of the harness so I ended up being the sled dog. Kalle pooped out pretty quickly though (she is riding on the sled, I am pulling it, and she is whining about being tired and wants to go home???) so we didn't actually find our tree yet. Maybe tomorrow. But it was beautiful out with soft fresh snow and very good cross country skiing!

MONDAY, DECEMBER 11, 2006
8:20 PM

Jaimi and Kevin arrived today! So we are gathered around en force again. I went to Portland to hit Costco and pick them up while Rob stayed home with Gene. Jill got his fluids started before she left for work, but Rob switched bags and disconnected him when done! That Rob, he can do anything. And Gene is feeling MUCH better today. Rob is good for him.

We had a nice family day yesterday. Rob cooked ham and scalloped potatoes and made a great fruit salad with ginger yogurt dressing. While the ham was cooking, Rob, Dillon, Ellie and I made another foray out after a tree and this time came home with one in tow. Rob paraded it by the living room window and got thumbs up from Gene, Juli and Jill but they admitted part of the approval might have been that they didn't have to go find it more than that it was a beautiful tree. It is a bit smaller than in the past years, probably only about 10 feet tall, but I was ready to settle for boughs on the stair rails, so it is looking pretty grand to me.

WEDNESDAY, DECEMBER 13, 2006
11:20 PM

Gene has been doing well this week! We even got him on the stair stepper for a few minutes yesterday. He doesn't have much stamina but we'll get him built back up.

Ellie came for the day yesterday. We have really missed our Tuesday and Thursday Ellie days so it is great to finally have some days home so we can have her! She, Kevin and I baked Christmas cookies, which Kevin, Kalle, Jaimi and I decorated after school today. After school yesterday, Jaimi, Kalle, Kevin and I got the tree up under Gene's close supervision (more to the right, no I mean left. . .) It was not the most beautiful tree ever, but it was up and decorated. Last night about 11:30, I heard a strange whoosh followed by jingling noise and went into the living room to find the tree lying over the back of the couch. Gene had heard it too, and hit the living room about the same time I did. I went and got Jaimi and Jill out of bed to help us get it back on its feet and remove most of the ornaments. I spent the whole time grumbling about how I KNEW we shouldn't bother with a tree this year and so on until Jaimi and Jill started calling me Eeyore.

We decided to leave it and just go buy a better tree today (we have not bought a tree since we moved

51

into this pine and fir forest we call a ranch). But this morning I decided we WOULD make this one work before I would go spend 40 bucks on a tree. Kevin told me he thought the tree fell over because all of the ornaments were on one side of the tree. I told him he had a point there, but it was necessary to do it that way because all of the boughs are on one side of the tree! Never-the-less we got it back up, wired it to the stair rail and redecorated it. Jill came home in the middle of this project and asked what happened to the idea of just buying a GOOD tree. Jaimi told her that when I announced we were fixing this one, it was so un-Eeyore-like that she figured she should just go with it.

Still not the best looking tree ever (and even not as good looking as before because the lights are hanging pretty chaotically after their fling to the floor), but lets hope it remains standing through the night! The funny part was that Gene was so casual about the whole thing that I finally told him that cancer must have made him mellow. He said it just helps you figure out what matters. Apparently not the Christmas tree laying over the back of the couch! And I guess not having the ugliest Christmas tree ever, either!

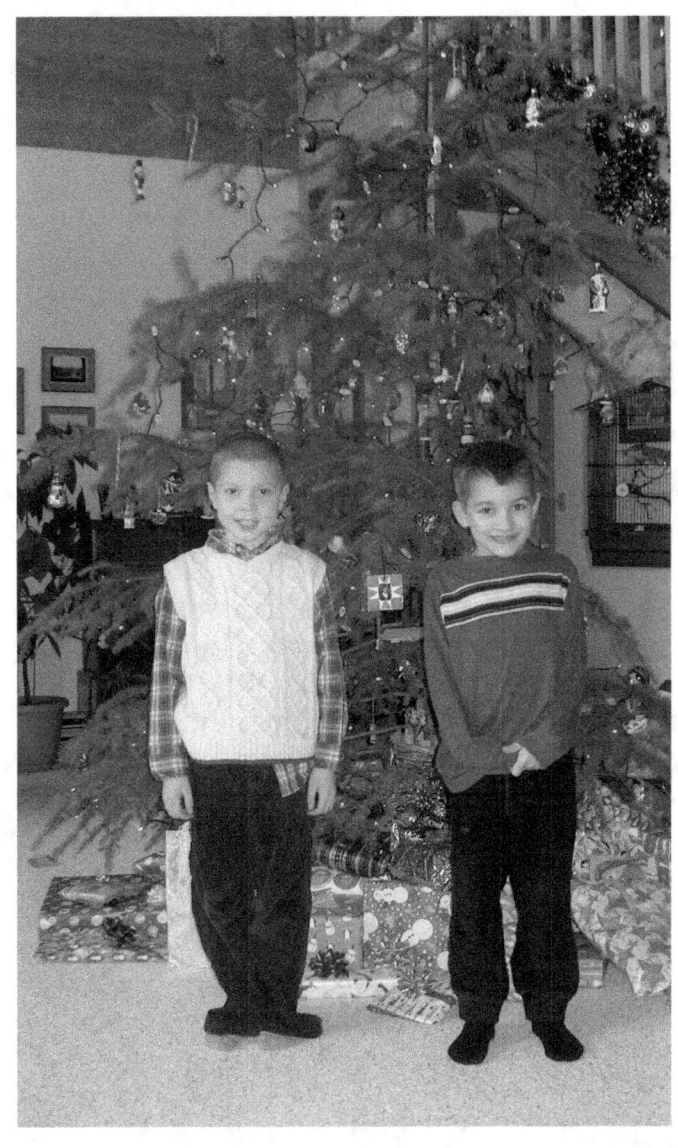

Dillon and Kevin standing dangerously close to the precarious Christmas tree:

Yes, Kevin, they're all on one side. . .

THURSDAY, DECEMBER 14, 2006
11:13 PM

I laughed when I read Fred's guest book entry about Gene being well-known.

Gene, I was reading Mike's entry and wanted to share that yes, you and your character are well known -- I was talking to Pat this week and he said he was at a convention and overheard your name being mentioned at a booth as he walked by and had to follow-up to see if there was another Gene Cyrus in the PNW. No, it was you -- it was some Philips/Heartstream folks talking about you! I'm sure it was good talk though.

His fame (or infamy) seems to keep cropping up in these entries. He's always had the ability to claim a total stranger as a friend within a few minute interaction, and seems like everywhere we go, we run into someone who knows Gene. But since I was only 17 when I married him, I just kind of took it for granted until one time around 1990, Gene went with an HP colleague and I on a business trip to Bristol, England. Daren, Gene and I were wandering around lost and Gene stopped to ask a local for directions. They visited a few minutes, then Gene came back to us with directions. As we were walking away, the guy yelled, "Hey, Gene!" He had thought of something else he needed to add, but Daren was amazed that he already knew Gene's name.

Later in the same trip, we spent a day in Lincoln. We took the train up from London, then Daren and I headed out to a vendors and left Gene to do some sight seeing. We agreed on a meeting time at a downtown pub. When we got back to the pub that afternoon, we walked in. No sign of Gene but there was a large crowd of people in the back of the pub. Daren and I looked at each other and said, "That would be Gene."

After awhile, the kids and I just started calling him "Hi I'm Gene." For his 50th birthday party (held in Panama so most of you missed it), we made name tags for everyone to wear, but they all said "Hi I'm Gene." The family wore ours on Hearstream shirts with the logo "HeartstreAM The Legend Lives On" only we put our name tags over the Heartstream part so they just read "Hi I'm Gene, The Legend Lives On". I wrote lyrics to Master of the House and the kids (who we called the Panamaniacs) performed it at the party. Here are some of the lyrics:

> *Master of the House, doling out the chores,*
> *Ready with a handshake ,*
> *And a pat on the bean.*
> *Tells a saucy tale, Makes a little stir*
> *Everyone appreciates "Hi I'm Gene!"*
> *Glad to do a friend a favor,*
> *Doesn't cost him to be nice*
> *But nothing gets you something,*
> *Only if you add a little spice.*
> *Master of the House, Keeper of the Zoo,*
> *Ready to call you a name or two.*
> *Calls you a dork, how can that be great,*
> *but he makes us feel good though we*
> *can't see straight.*
> *Everyone loves the turkey,*

Everybody's bosom friend.

He's really an old geezer

But 50 years is clearly not the end.

Master of the House, Keeper of the zoo,

He's been Mr. Mom and the Pool Boy, too.

He talks to the dogs, sets the kids straight,

He's a lot of fun and a lifelong mate.

When it comes to cleaning barns,

Or knocking down big trees,

Greeting strangers like he knows them,

How it all increases,

this is the legend that is Gene.

From the Guestbook:

THURSDAY, DECEMBER 14, 2006

I'm gonna have to stop watching reruns. This isn't the one I said I'd send, but its in my head now so I might as well send it:

(Beverly Hillbillies theme song)

Come and listen to a story bout a man named Gene.

A real cool dude always kept his whiskers clean.

Then one day while driving into town,

up from his chest came a terrible sound.

Cancer that is, Scary Staff, the Big C.

Well, first thing ya know Gene's in the doctor's chair.

Kin folk said "Gene, you're gonna lose your hair!

Said chemotherapy is what is best for you.

So he loaded up his spunk and did what he had to do.

Treatment, that is. Chemo drips, CT Scans.

So now its time for all to pray for Gene and his kin.

And they would like to thank you folks for kindly droppin in.

Don't forget to drop a line at this locality.
With our help, he'll beat this thing, I think you'll all agree.
Ya All Come back now, ya hear.
Big Al

MONDAY, DECEMBER 18, 2006
1:25 PM

We had a big storm Thursday night and Rob got called out for work at 9:30. I think he finally got home again Friday night about midnight, then back to work at 6 am. And it continues like that still. So Rob missed Family Day this week. And bummer cuz it was spectacular. Apparently the girls decided Gene would be too sick after chemo this week to really enjoy Christmas, so he got to open some presents yesterday. They included some warm slippers and a BMW.

WHAT???? Yes, indeed, a red BMW X5 (small SUV). The girls thought the old Suburban (with 185,000 miles on it) was just getting too rickety and uncomfortable for the sick guy to ride in, so Jaimi and Jill drove it to Yakima yesterday and came back with the new car (and brought the salesman home for dinner). It is WAY COOL!

So we were excited to head off to Celilo this morning in a shiny COMFY car. However, Dr. Taylor checked Gene out and sent him home for another week. He weighed in at 124 pounds and the doc is afraid chemo this week would have bottomed him out so told him to rest and eat another week and come back for more next week. In the meantime, he decided to do another CT scan

57

(Wed) to see if we are beating the thing--I think he would love to not have to take Gene the whole four rounds.

So more news later this week, hopefully.

SATURDAY, DECEMBER 23, 2006
3:58 PM

Gosh, it has been a really busy week. I'm not sure how we would have fit chemo in so guess it is good it got postponed. Of course, even when we are home, about half the day gets used up running the fluids, so with dark coming around 4, the days are pretty short.

Wednesday we did the CT scan and believe it or not, Gene managed almost the entire two bottles of Berry Smoothie! No results yet. We did not insist on a CD this time so I have not been able to look at it. I called Dr. Taylor's office yesterday but they did not have the radiologists report yet and had not looked at it themselves. So we will just have to sit on our hands till Tuesday when we will see Dr. Taylor and can get the scoop. In the meantime, Gene has had a very good week with only a few upsets. I think he has put on about 5 pounds so that is very good. We had visits from Chuck, Kimmy, Doug and Esther this week. For awhile Gene really did not feel like visitors but he enjoyed the company this week since he felt so much better.

Thanks for great dinners this week from church friends Sharon, Lynn, Shirley and Lynette, and Deborah and a chocolate cake to die for from Vida at Kalle's school. We felt a little guilty eating

58

so well on non-chemo week (dinners were scheduled based on EXPECTING chemo) but we did squirrel away half of the enchiladas and half the chicken casserole for next week.

I had a hectic day yesterday: got Gene started with his fluids then left Jaimi in charge while the girls and I took the garbage to the dump (OH MY GOODNESS, where does all that come from???? My truck was FULL), got gas, picked up the groceries for Christmas Eve supper, dropped of a gift for Dr. Sherpa, got a couple bales of straw and mineral blocks for the horses and made a quick stop at Juli's shop for some scrap booking stuff to finish the gifts I was making the girls. While I was running around, Jaimi called to tell me some people wanted to come look at ponies. Doug and Esther were scheduled for 2:00 but I told Jaimi I definitely needed to let the pony lookers come, so she called them back and told them to come at 2:30. I got home about 1:00, unloaded, grabbed half a sandwich, then Breanna and I quickly rode a couple of ponies. Since none of them have been ridden since all this started in October, I wasn't about to put someone else's kids on them without checking them out. They were good as gold though. Then I ran in the house to drink a glass of wine with our friends, then back out to show ponies. The people stayed till dark, so then it was chores and eat up the yummy soup Deborah sent, get Kalle a bath and off to bed. Then I spent till midnight finishing my little gift project (I am SO proud of myself: I'll tell y'all next week what I made!)

We woke up this morning to 5 or 6 inches of snow. After "drinking" his saline and potassium, Gene bundled up and pulled the kids on the sleds with his tractor. He has gotten out of the house a lot more this week. It is so good to see him more active. I guess that will screech to a halt again next week though!

Tomorrow is Christmas Eve. Juli and family will join the rest of us up here at the ranch. They always sleep over on Christmas Eve even though they live in town because Juli wants to wake up with the whole family on Christmas morning. Rob must think we are a weird bunch but he humors us all. We are hoping Gene will feel good enough to go to church (he doesn't go out in public much because he looks a little funny hauling around his puke buckets) but if not maybe we will all just sing some carols by candlelight here. No one really wants to go off and leave him alone on Christmas Eve! Gene with the queasy stomach has blessed the scrapping of the Oyster Stew tradition for this year so it is Raclette and Jaimi's basil soup for Christmas Eve, then she is making her famous peppercorn lamb for Christmas dinner.

We have not sent out our Christmas letters, which is not even unusual since I never get it done before New Year's anyway, but this year in particular, we want you all to know how thankful we are for your love and support. We wish you all a blessed Christmas and pray we will ALL come into a better and healthier new year. Merry Christmas!

TUESDAY, DECEMBER 26, 2006
2:29 PM

I know a lot of people are anxiously awaiting the update on Gene's doctor's appointment today, so I will get right to it and then tell you about our Christmas festivities.

We got to Celilo about 8:30 this morning and Dr. Taylor came right in to let us know that the cat scan shows the lung tumor continues to shrink and in fact has now separated away from the lung wall. This actually means it would be operable except since there are mets we have to continue with chemo to eradicate them anyway so not much point in taking out the lung mass. The liver mets are still visible but also are shrinking, so all-in-all, very good news. He also decided to do a trial run of bleomycin with the hopes of replacing the ifosfomide he has been using with bleomycin which is more specific for germ cell tumors. He has put it off until now because it can be hard on the lungs and since Gene had received a number of radiation treatments prior to the germ cell diagnosis, wanted to give the lung some recovery time first. If there are no adverse reactions to the bleomycin, Gene will be getting it once a week and continue the last two cycles of 1 week on and 2 weeks off with the other 2 drugs (etoposide and cisplatin).

So the big question remaining is "are we winning" and the conditional answer to that is that everything is going in the right direction. In about 3 months time they will repeat the PET scan to see if there are any remaining or recurring viable cancer cells but at this time all we know is that things are shrinking. Since the entire middle of the big tumor was pretty much dead when detected, it is possible that it is already pretty much killed but no way to tell for sure except by taking it out, which he is not inclined to do. And in the meantime we will have periodic cat scans to monitor the size of the tumors.

61

The dead stuff should at some point start breaking up and get recycled by the body.

Our Christmas was great, thanks to Gene's extra week off. He was feeling pretty darn good and that definitely contributed to a happy mood all around. I had been dreading Christmas a little, thinking about faking good cheer and fun but it turned out to be real after all. I was a little worried about Christmas morning though because 2 days before, my latte machine bit the dust and went on the load to the dump.

Christmas Eve, the Risings arrived shortly after noon. We had a mid-afternoon "supper" of Jaimi's cream of basil soup with cherry tomatoes and our traditional Raclette (minus the Raclette. . .) Then we ALL (yup--Gene's first outing in a couple of months!) went to the 5:00 Christmas Eve service at our church. Afterwards we came home and had champagne while the kids opened presents, then put them to bed and got to the serious business of our crazy gift exchange. I drew the low number and chose the heaviest gift, which turned out to be dumbbells and pilate bands (meant for Gene but close enough). When it was Gene's turn, he chose what turned out to be a Starbucks latte machine! Of course, my next turn around, I stole that baby right out from under him. I know, he probably would have let me use it but wouldn't the girls have been disappointed if I hadn't stolen it??? I think next year we might have to put a price limit on the gift exchange but boy are we all thankful for that latte machine! Other than the latte machine and Jaimi's basil soup, the highlight of the evening was Rob's ceviche. Steve and Anita, you would have been impressed. Every bit as good as the Shell station in Panama City!

After a largely sleepless night (Juli says Kalle snores louder than Steve!) and a very early start (thanks a lot, Dillon and Kalle!) we had the Christmas morning fun of seriously overflowing stockings and Santa toys. We all played in our jammies till dinner time, then enjoyed Jaimi's famous peppercorn encrusted leg of lamb. Then we topped off the fun with our place marker "crackers". If you don't know what they are, we make them by filling cardboard tubes with toys, candies, lip gloss, charms or whatever, stringing a pull-apart fire cracker through the middle, wrapping it in wrapping paper and tying the ends of the firecracker to ribbons on each end so when you pull the paper apart, the fire cracker goes off, shooting the treasures inside all over. Jill was in charge of inserting the charade cards and also took upon herself to write a family Christmas poem which got read around the table (and therefore out of order but even more fun) prior to charades. The poem began with "Twas the night before Christmas and all through the house, not a creature was stirring, not even a louse" and ended with "We wish you a Merry Christmas, we wish you a Merry Christmas, we wish you a Merry Christmas and a lot of new hair." so you can see it is in competition with some of Al's finer contributions!

We were sad to see the day end but were energized and ready for this new week of chemo.

FRIDAY, DECEMBER 29, 2006
7:51 PM

It's now Friday morning, and we are on second-to-last chemo day of this cycle. I've been "on duty" the past 3 days (this is Jaimi), and since tomorrow mom is back on, it just may be my last chemo run altogether! I probably won't be in town for the next cycle, so I certainly hope this is it, and next time I'm here it's to celebrate licking the beast!

Sitting here watching dad sleep, I'm feeling in higher spirits than yesterday. After a night of really poor sleep, dad was in pretty bad shape yesterday. So I sat here anxiously trying to keep myself busy while he sat/slept/sicked and generally looked miserable. Thank goodness for little inconveniences like stock market shifts and bank accounts not set up properly, so I have a few mundane things to worry about and keep from worrying about the big things! He did get the full bleomycin dose yesterday and it seemed to go in okay, so we are hopeful this will be the heavy-duty artillery to finish off the cancer war.

Last night, dad did okay eating again at least, but after a couple iffy days he is back down 5 pounds to 126 today. At least he slept better last night, so he looks and is a lot more alert. And he got his superman steroid, so hopefully that will also help put some bounce back in his step. He managed to converse a bit with me before taking a nap, and I've felt good enough about how he's doing to go down to the spa for a shower and I'll head out to do a bit of shopping in a minute. Yesterday I was afraid to venture out for a cup of tea! So, it's a good day.

Hope you all have had great holidays - thanks for the continued wishes and prayers. We sure appreciate it, and it is great to see things start to come together in a positive direction!

SATURDAY, DECEMBER 30, 2006
7:25 PM

Today was the last day in this chemo cycle. Since Monday was Christmas day, we started the five day cycle on Tuesday so today we went to the hospital in The Dalles instead of the Celilo Center. It was not quite as organized. The front desk didn't know we were coming so we had to get over the "how do we bill you if we don't know you are here" issues before we could finally get to a room. Turns out the nurse didn't actually know we were coming either so killed a little more time while she talked to the pharmacist who did know we were coming and in fact had the very organized package of fluids and drugs as delivered by the Celilo pharmacist and called one of the Celilo nurses for advice. After that, she got Gene hooked up and very efficiently and cheerfully got him through the day. He felt pretty good and ate a turkey sandwich for lunch then ate firsts AND seconds of chicken, beans and cantaloupe for dinner. So all-in-all he finished out this chemo week a little better than the last.

Life is a Journey, not a Destination

Today is New Year's Eve. Probably the most celebrated night of the year. A time to celebrate the year behind us, plan and look forward to the new year ahead. 2006 has in many ways been one of the hardest in our lives, so it seems like we might just say, "Whew, glad that's over." And get on with 2007. But, in fact, we have much to celebrate and oddly enough, much of it is related to the dastardly journey we are in the midst of. Truly, it is not a journey that we would have chosen to take, but like lots of the hard things in life, it does have its silver linings as well. And most of that is related to you, the people reading this, who in one way or another have chosen to carry us a step or three along the way.

If you have ever been to a training session led by Gene, you likely have heard the analogy he uses, referring to life as a train ride. Our friend, Bud, recently sent us a link to a website that has made this analogy into a flash movie. It is a beautiful and meaningful internet "movie" about how people get on and off the train ride of our lives, some for only a short time and some for the whole ride. It seemed so appropriate since Gene has used this story many times and because it is so germane to this journey we are on and the ties and rails each of you have laid before us to help us through. Something I have learned on this journey is that pretty much anyone who has ever ridden the train with Gene has come back to help keep him on the ride. It is both a complement to him as a person and a symbol of how good he is at choosing friends!

I have mentioned before that Gene keeps worrying about whether I have answered all the messages and greetings coming in the way of guest book entries, emails, cards and phone calls and I have admitted not keeping up very well with it. But we are so grateful for all these words of support, as well as the food, help with chores, and prayers coming from so many directions. So my New Year's celebration is to celebrate each of you.

Gene and I won't be out partying tonight. Actually, I have to admit that we almost never party on New Year's Eve so this won't be a huge break from tradition. But we feel like we truly have something to celebrate even in the midst of puke buckets and hydration IVs and we thank you all for this. Thanks for being with us on our life's journey!

THURSDAY, JANUARY 04, 2007
10:35 PM

Well, what next?

Remember Juli complaining about not being able to sleep cuz of Kalle's snoring? Well, it just kept getting worse, so I got a flashlight and looked down her throat and sure enough: her tonsils were kissing. She has always sounded like she had adenoid problems and last summer her tonsils looked a little large, so we took her in to an ear, nose and throat doc for a check. He said they were a little large but it was really borderline as to whether she should have them out so of course we opted not to do it. Bad plan I guess. I took her back today and he said, "These have to come out. How about Tuesday? (his next surgery day)" She sounds so bad now (she even snores when she's awake) that I asked him if I should worry about them strangling her in the meantime. He said no, unless she were to get sick in which case they might swell even more and then she could be in trouble. They are really huge! great timing, huh?

Kalle, interestingly, is thrilled beyond belief. She is going around having happy seizures all over the place. Why? Well, 1) she heard she gets all the ice cream she wants 2) She thinks she will have a girly voice afterwards (kids tease her that she has a boy voice because it is so low), 3) she will get to crawl in bed with mom and dad again (when she comes down at night now, I take her back up to her bed cuz she snores so loud Dad wouldn't get any sleep, and 4) she gets to miss school for a week or so. Oh to be a child again!

Meanwhile, Gene weighed in at a mighty 124.6 today when he went for his bleo blast. He is still staying pretty close to the puke buckets but is definitely having a better week after this cycle than last. Hopefully he will be feeling pretty good next week as I move to my new caregiver role. . .

Now to the important stuff: Al, it doesn't matter how long your new verse is. The world wants to see it. Load away!

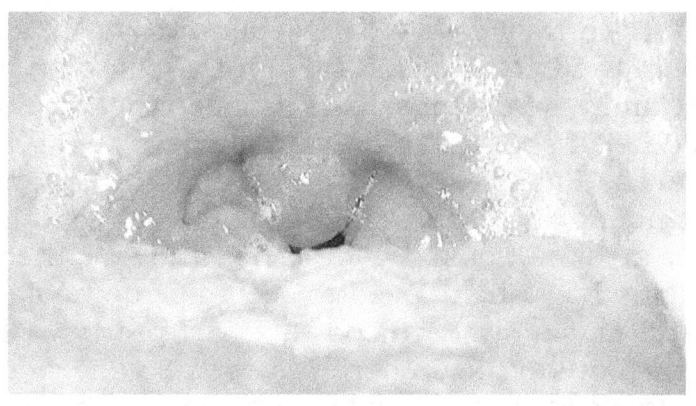

Kalle's tonsils

TUESDAY, JANUARY 09, 2007
10:19 PM

Yesterday we started getting ready for the big tonsil day by going to the drug store to pick up Kalle's pain medicine. Ruth, from our church, was there and gave her a purple poodle to take to the hospital! We got home, had dinner and bath and got into bed pretty early.

Kalle woke up at 5:30 this morning ready to go get her tonsils out. I stuck her in bed with Gene while I got dressed and fed horses, then we loaded up and headed for The Dalles. We got there right on time at 7:30, got her into the hospital jammies and both had back massages while we waited our turn. A little after 8:00, Nurse Brian took us down to the surgery ward. We sat in a little room till the anesthesiologist talked to us, then the tonsil doctor stuck his head in to say hi. He was already in his surgical garb and Kalle said, "Hey, you look good in that hat, it brings out your eyes." He looked a little shocked but then laughed and said that's what all the girls say.

Then they gave me a beeper and took Kalle away to the OR. She said they put stickers on her chest and a space mask on her face. Then they asked her if she had a dog and she told them his name was Fletcher and that is the last thing she remembers until she woke up. Then she saw the IV in her arm and looked behind her and saw the medicine bag (she is used to seeing Gene hooked up for fluids so understood this part pretty well) but she couldn't keep her eyes open so she went back to sleep. Then they brought her on the bed back up to me. She woke up on the way up and was kind of disoriented and upset that her throat hurt so she needed a bit more medicine, a back rub and a lullaby and then went back to sleep for about an hour. She was much friendlier when she woke up the next time, but wanted to go home real bad. She said she changed her mind and getting tonsils out is not so fun after-all. Finally about noon they kicked us out. Kalle got a wheelchair ride to the car which she thought was pretty cool and we drove home to Daddy.

Daddy, by the way, was home alone. Even more shocking is that he took the girls to school before returning home to be home alone. After three weeks of having Jaimi here, and Juli off work, and Jill around, we were suddenly on our own with Jaimi gone, Jill gone (get this: Jaimi was already back in the US in Las Vegas for a conference so Jill flew down for a couple of days), and Juli back at work. So luckily it was on Gene's good week (back to chemo NEXT week)!

When Kalle and I got home, I got her settled on the love seat, then got Gene-on the couch-hooked up for his fluids and the living room was just full of patients and puke buckets. Juli picked the girls up along with dinner (an amazing looking rice dish with big chunks of carrots and thick slices of turkey breast on top, fruit salad and chocolate torte!) from Deborah, popsicles from Kalle's teacher, and a bear and balloon from Ellie and Dillon. By then Kalle had eaten ice cream a couple of times, drunk some very cold apple juice, and was deciding maybe it wasn't all so bad again. She has been up and down a few times since then, depending on how long it has been since the pain medicine.

I'm sure you are all enjoying today's pre-op picture of Kalle's mouth and throat!

TUESDAY, JANUARY 09, 2007

THE DUDE ON THE BIKE
By Big Al
Twas the night before Christmas
And all through the Ranch
Hope had not faded
No way, not a chance.
The tree was lashed
To the stairwell with wire
The chimney was hot
From the freshly built fire
The kids were all sleeping
Wherever they fell
They worried about Papa
Who was going through Hell.
And Mama in here jama's
And Papa in his chair
Had just settled down
To count what was left of his hair.
When out in the woods
There arose such a noise
That everyone woke
All the girls, All the boys
They peered through the drapes
And the doors and the like
And stared at this Dude
On a strange looking bike
What the heck is that
Papa said under his breath.
That guy looks just awful
Like warmed over death.
The Dude just stared back at them
Nodding his head
His hair all tangled
His eyes bloodshot red
The children were frightened
As well as they should
They had no idea
If he was bad or was good
They all ran to Papa
Who opened his arms
And calmed them by saying
There was no need for alarm.
That Dude wants me to go
But you have to be steady

72

I'll tell him no way
That I'll go when I'm ready
So he opened the door
And walked out on the deck
Strolled up to the Dude
Who looked like a wreck
The Dude spoke to Papa
And told him the truth
You're not the same person
You were in your youth
You were given this test
That God knew you could take
But your faith just grew stronger
Which is good for your sake
God sees that you're needed
Much more here at home
They all need you more
Even that guy that writes poems
You've lived your life well
God wants you to know
A reward is all yours
For the faith that you show
So you go to the Doctors
And do what they say
And soon that lung tumor
Will just go away
Then the Dude stood straight up
Must have been seven feet tall
And nodded his head
As if to say, "That's All"
Then he turned on his bike
And without any sound
He vanished, leaving Papa
Just looking around
So Papa went back
Inside the ranch
And looked at an Angel
Hanging on a tree branch
The family gathered round
With tears in their eyes
They all hugged dear Papa
All courageous and wise
He told them what happened
Outside with the Dude
And pointed to the Angel
To brighten their mood
He said Angels come in
All shapes and sizes
That Dude on the Bike

73

Was one of the wisest
He was sent here by God
To give us good news
He said that my family
Was too precious to lose
So their tears turned to joy
Such good news he had
There no longer was
Any reason to be sad
That's the story of Dude
And Papa and All
That night in the woods
Snow starting to fall
When Faith saved a Papa
And Hope proved its might
Merry Christmas to All
And to All a Good Night!

FRIDAY, JANUARY 12, 2007
10:35 PM

Okay, so Juli didn't like the tonsil picture. I, myself, was quite proud of it. Oh well. So to keep Juli happy, I put the good picture of Gene back up. It is appropriate to do this today because. . . [drum roll] . . . he is growing new hair! I was shocked and amazed that he would be getting new hair while he is still doing chemo, but maybe the drug they switched out (Ifosfomide for bleomycin) was the hair culprit because indeed there are tiny baby hairs coming in all over his head. Can't tell what color they are yet, but I am hoping for grey cuz it isn't fair that I should be the only grey one after all this.

It has been a rough week. I sort of figured Kalle would not be a great patient but in fact, the first three days she felt so awful she barely moved. We just felt bad for her and did a lot of lap time. But she does not take medicine well; getting the pain meds down was next to impossible so we

74

couldn't do much to make her feel better. Today, after a rough night, she slept until noon then late this afternoon perked up enough to become a horrible monster. She has not taken her Risperdal for 3 days (cuz I can't get her to drink enough of anything to get it down) and I guess you could say she needs it. . . I finally got nearly a full dose down her tonight so hopefully she will be a little tamer tomorrow. We will have to get her back on an even keel before sending her back to school!

I got the farrier set up for Monday so I can get horse feet trimmed, especially Tierney as he heads to Canada for a new home next week. I am sad to see him go; he was my horse show buddy last year and one of my favorites. But I need to sell ponies so gotta sell what the buyer wants. Anyway, while talking to Jackie, I found out she has some guys who do work for them so I asked if I could hire them away for a bit to get my hay moved. We put about ten tons of hay up where we were building the new barn, expecting to have half the horses moved up there this winter. Well, those plans all came to a screeching halt in October, so that hay has been sitting up there molding under the tarp and meanwhile I am running out here. So I have a little crew coming on Sunday to get the hay (whatever is left good in the middle) moved over here. I drove up to the barn today to make sure we could get in. The guy who did the road never finished the job so when it is wet, you can't get in. If you are thinking of doing any excavation or road work around here, call me to find out who NOT to hire! The good news about the cold weather is that it is frozen instead of wet, but thought I better be sure it was frozen enough that the guys wouldn't get stuck. I have not been up to the barn in many weeks; I avoid going up there because it depresses me. I had no problem getting in and out; it is pretty frozen, but I found that the guy who was working on the office and tack room left the job without battening down the hatches so the doors were not properly latched. One of them blew off in the big wind. The door is demolished and it also ripped out some of the trim. So that was a particularly depressing trip; the crappy road, my poor abandoned half finished barn, hay molding under a tarp because we never got it moved into the barn, and a poor bent door stuck in the mud in the breezeway. I came home bawling my head off and hid under the covers in the bed but Gene caught me anyway. He pointed out that in the scheme of things, it is not a big deal. Nothing else is really a big deal when you are fighting cancer, but then on the other hand, when you are emotionally wiped out, everything seems like a big deal even if it isn't. If I am honest, I guess, the really big deal to me wasn't the door, it was the whole thing of starting the dream barn and then abandoning it and just wishing we had never sunk that much money into it because I don't know if we will ever finish it and we could be paying bills with all that money. So anyway, really no big deal but a big "pity party" anyway.

Seems like Fridays are bad days for me. Who came up with the TGIF stuff?

But Gene has hair. Almost.

Well, we are almost finished with the next to last day of the last chemo cycle! Gene has done really well this week. He was great Monday and Tuesday, then things got a little rocky from there, but he is getting through it. About 2 weeks from now we should be ready for a big celebration. He will continue to have the once a week bleo treatment about 3 more times but the horrible 5 day in a row treatment will end tomorrow!

Kalle went back to school today. It was rough but she finally got through the real hurty part and was pretty much back to normal yesterday. I took her to McDonalds Tuesday but the chicken nuggets still hurt her throat so that turned out to not be such a treat after all. She has enjoyed the big box of popsicles her teacher sent her and ate all the little ice cream cups I bought, but that only after the third day or so. Those first few days she pretty much couldn't eat or drink anything!

But the snoring is gone! And she is thrilled when we tell her she has a girly giggle now.

My pony, Tierney, is being picked up as we speak. I could not get home in time so the hauler was going to pick Jill up at the vet clinic so she can make sure they get the right horse, paperwork, etc. I am sad not to see him off, but on the other hand, maybe it's better this way.

Monday Juli brought Gene to chemo and I stayed home to help move hay. The to-be-hired boys were no shows, but Matt (our farrier) and his son Nick did it. We saved probably about 3 tons out

77

of about 10. The Eeyore in me is depressed, but the new improved Gene is very philosophical about its importance in the overall scheme of things. But I better call Ken and make sure he will have some more hay for me come March cuz I am gonna run out!

This has been a sort of weird chemo week. Juli took Gene on Monday. Tuesday, he took himself! He thought Kalle should stay home which that meant I should stay home, so that left him to drive himself. Jill offered to take off work, but he insisted on going alone. And he did just fine, still felt pretty good till Wednesday morning. Wednesday Kalle and I took him in and hung out a little, then went over to her doctor for her follow-up check and release to go back to school, then we worked on homework and went shopping, and out to lunch.

So today was my first day to just do "normal" chemo day stuff. I hung out with Gene for awhile till he was all hooked up and settled in, then I went down to the spa, enjoyed the hot tub, took a shower (and washed my hair with lotion--oh well, those darn bottles all look the same!), then went back up and had a back massage while I sat with Gene till my friend Marilyn came to take me to lunch. Yeah, I know, chemo days sound a lot more fun for me than for Gene. But when we left him, his chicken soup was on order and he was getting a foot massage, so that is not all bad either!

Juli is busily planning Dillon's second annual birthday party at the beach. After Jaimi's stunning performance as the lead ballerina at Ellie's Twelve Dancing Princesses party in December, Juli is lobbying for her to come back for Dillon's:

78

Jaimi,

Can you guys make it for Dillon's birthday? We are celebrating it, and dad's end of CHEMO, at the BEACH, at the Beach Dream house!!! We are going Friday February16th till the 19th. We know you just left, but you must admit it's tempting. Dillon wants to know why Kevin always comes for Ellie's birthday, and not his! :) Also, can you do an under the sea dance, dressed as sponge bob???;)

Dad's last day of chemo was a long one, especially since the nurses called MY cell phone after mom & dad had left Celilo, 20 minutes prior, because a nurse had forgotten, "a very important shot" so mom & dad had to turn around (after I called twice to no answer on mom's cell) and go back to Celilo!

WHEEWee, didn't think I could get that story out! It is late, just got back from midnight madness, I had to put it on by myself :(and really missed mom & Jill (and YOU Jaimi) but at least I got home before 2 in the morning. It was a great group of ladies, but nothing as exciting as safari albums tonight! Guess I'd better go to bed! Yay Dad!!! We are so proud of you for making it through these grueling months! And can't wait for you to get back to your endearing, 150 pound, obnoxious, hairy, dork calling, self!!! I'll bet you'll start feeling better just in time for LOST, and don't forget, Prison Break starts THIS Monday! And by Beach trip weekend you'll be up for anything!!!

Love you Guys! You are the SUNS in my shine!

Jules

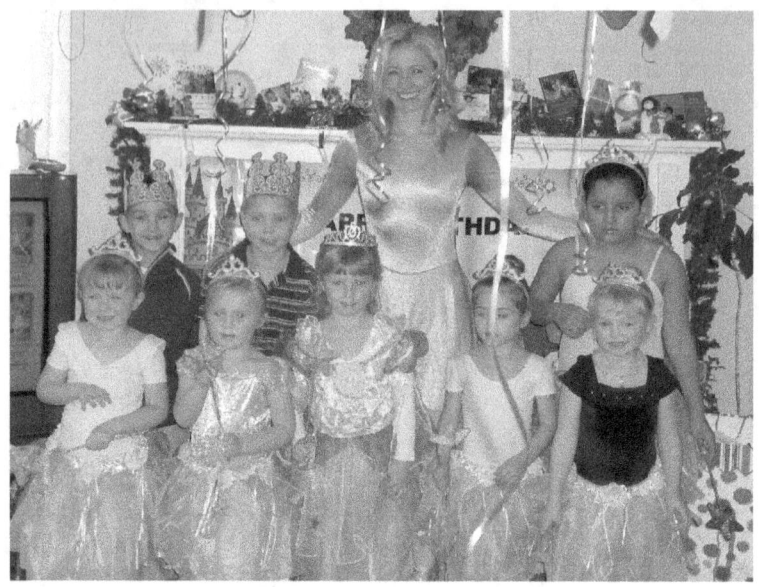

Well, guess I'll run back up and see if the last bag has finished so I can take my chemo boy home.

WEDNESDAY, JANUARY 24, 2007
11:26 AM

It's Wednesday and we are back at Celilo for the bleo treatment. This happens today and next Wednesday, then on Feb 5 we go in for another CT scan. So we will be anxiously waiting for that day!

Meanwhile, Gene is slowly starting to feel a bit better after his big week of chemo last week. Hopefully, by the weekend he will be feeling well enough to get out for a small walk. He is still very tired and weak, but I could tell he was beginning to perk up a bit when I overheard him and Kalle having a big long heart to heart Monday night. He has always been Kalle's confidante; she tells him way more than she will me about what is going on at school, etc. Last year when he was in Atlanta, she would have to call him every day to talk about Maddie. Maddie is one of Kalle's friends, a very nice little girl, but last year the boy Kalle liked was more interested in Maddie than Kalle and she was having a hard time with the green eyed monster. She would talk to Gene every night about what she would LIKE to do to Maddie and Gene would try to help her find ways to feel better. Yes, Kalle was only 8. I can't wait until she is a teenager!

One good part of this whole ordeal (for me at least) is that she has started talking to me more about things. Last week she was not happy about going back to school and said it was because Coby always makes ugly faces at her. She said that Julia, Coby's cousin, told Kalle he was just playing, but she did not think it was nice at all. I told her maybe she could tell Coby she did not like it and ask him to play some other way. Kalle said, "Mom, you just don't understand bullies in this century." I guess my age is showing. . .

Speaking of Kalle, she has recovered completely. She had a great day at school yesterday and even got two treats for good work. The only post-tonsillectomy downside is that she is sleeping so much better than she needs less of it. I actually liked putting her to bed at 7:30 and hearing her snore within minutes. Now she is still squirming around till 8 or 9:00.

Matt came over and got a little more than half the horses feet trimmed yesterday, so Ellie and I had some outdoor time helping with that. It was a little crazy running back and forth to check on Gene's IVs but luckily Matt is very easy going and just goes with the flow. After the horses were done,

81

Ellie and I made raspberry tarts and chocolate pie. I have missed my Ellie days so it is nice to be getting back to a little more normal routine and getting time with her again. Hopefully tomorrow we will have time to get her pony out for awhile!

WEDNESDAY, JANUARY 31, 2007
4:22 PM

Leslie (Gene's sister) has been complaining about the lack of updates. Okay, Les, I'm on it. I'm just afraid of boring everyone with the family journal thing since the health topic is pretty much samo samo (you know, puke buckets, etc.) But today is a big celebration day! Last day of chemo. Monday is the CT scan and Wednesday blood tests and doctor's appointment. So it will really be Wednesday before we have real news. Then hopefully it is hasta la vista to the cancer clinic for a little while and time to just build the boy back up! And hopefully toss those puke buckets into the recycling!

Other big deals in our lives this week: Friday is the funeral for our long time church pianist/organist. She was a charter member of the church and played nearly every Sunday until recently when she semi retired at ninety-something. She also served as council secretary as long as we have been there, maybe forever, I don't know. What a life of service! And a truly interesting and precious woman. We will miss her! Also Friday is our friend Sandi's CT scan. Please keep her in your prayers!

Not such a big deal, but good news: I found more hay AND the guy said he can deliver it. Wow! He can't stack it but will dump it in front of our hay tent and hopefully our neighbors Connor and Mark can help move it in. On second thought, I guess this IS a very big deal to 17 hungry horses (anyone want to buy a horse??? www.dancingmountainranch.com !)

Ellie and I made chocolate chip cookies Tuesday and she wondered how butter gets made. So we bought some cream and tomorrow we are making butter, and of course some biscuits to eat it on! It was not very nice weather to get outside, but we did manage to go out and lead Little Big Mac and pick up his feet. He will get his first hoof trim on Friday and I have hardly touched the poor boy since October so thought I better make sure he still remembered some of his early training. He did great so hopefully all will go well.

I know it is gauche to talk about money, but one day this may be a book and if anyone reads it who is going through what we are, this is sort of advice. First, I can't imagine how anyone could go through cancer by themselves. It seems like life should just leave you alone and let you get through it, but that never happens. The bills keep coming, the kids get sick, the hay rots and on top of that you are sick. And on top of all that are all these HUGE and mostly mysterious medical bills. We did not get many for awhile because everything gets submitted to the insurance first. But when they started coming it was in droves. We pretty much get 2 or 3 insurance "statement of benefits" a day. Then come the doctor's bills and those are usually pretty easy to figure out what you owe. THEN come the cancer center bills and boy oh boy, that is where you need some help! Once a month we get a bill from the medical center. It has a list of charges which are not described in any way except by the date they were billed to the insurance company. Then you look at the insurance company statements and they give treatment dates and the dates they processed the claim. So the only way to match the insurance benefits to the medical center bill is to try to find charge amounts that match. Can you imagine how hard that is when there are nearly a hundred of them???? But you gotta do it, because when I did the first months, I found two amounts that were billed in error so the insurance had not paid as much as they should have which means we were being billed more than we should have had to pay, charges that had not been preauthorized by the medical center so the insurance had not paid the full covered amount because it was not preauthorized (guess what, sometimes you can get stuff POST authorized and resubmit the bill and they will pay!), a number of charges the medical center showed but which had not been processed by the insurance company because they never got them??? Guess what, if they never get them it just looks like you owe the whole amount on the bottom line!, and finally, the worst of the worst, expenses that the insurance does not cover AT ALL! Don't you wish you knew what THOSE were in advance??? In our case, they denied the Neulasta shots (immune system booster given after each round of chemo). Gene needed four of them and they cost $6000 each. And the insurance company said they were not medically necessary so they wouldn't pay them. That had me awake nights! Well, you can also argue about that kind of stuff. In the end, the pharmacist wrote a letter explaining why it was medically necessary and that without them, Gene probably would have ended up in the hospital after each round of chemo at a much higher cost than the $6000 per shot and sure enough, they reversed the decision and are covering them, though I have not seen how much; hopefully it's covered like hospital costs and not like Rx costs which we get to pay half of.

Anyway, my advice is, if you ever have a major medical battle, first, make a spreadsheet with all the bills. I have one that shows treatment date, charge, what the insurance pays, and what we owe. I then gray out the cells when I get the medical center bills showing the matching amounts and when I pay what we owe, I gray that cell out. So it is easy (well, sort of) to make sure we are really only paying what I agree we owe. Otherwise, if you just pay what the medical center bills you for, you have no way of knowing if it is really right. I hit on this plan when I got the first bill and spent a couple hours on the phone with their billing department trying to figure out how to correlate it all. I did that in a panic when the bottom line on the bill showed WE owed them over $9,000 after only a few weeks worth of bills had run through the insurance! By the time I was done, the billing department and I agreed we owed $1900 at that point. Kind of a difference, huh??? And when I send a payment, I include a note saying what treatment dates I am paying for and I NEVER pay for any that I haven't gotten an insurance benefit statement for. Those ones I call up the billing department and tell them to resubmit the bill to insurance.

So, boring to most of you but maybe all that will help someone some day.

WEDNESDAY, FEBRUARY 07, 2007
6:41 PM

Hi Everyone, I know you are all anxiously awaiting this update so it will probably be a little anti-climatic to you as to us. The CT scan and doc visit went pretty much as expected. The scan shows the tumors continue to shrink but they are not gone. This is not necessarily bad news; the tissue appears very dense, which suggests they have been stripped of their blood supply and may in fact, be dead tissue. No way to tell that from the CT scan. The tumor markers (the blood tests that were the original basis for the germ cell diagnosis) have been looking good, but the counts from today's draw won't be available for a few days.

The good news is that Dr. Taylor has now decided to move up the date for the PET scan. Earlier he had said probably three months down the road, but now he has scheduled it for six weeks from now. So we won't have to wait as long to find out if there are any viable cancer cells left!

We had a great weekend. Friday I had five tons of hay delivered and dumped in the driveway in front of the hay tent, so Saturday, Gene drove the tractor while Rob, Juli, Jill, Dori, Breanna and I loaded and stacked the hay. Later, our friends, Dan, Carol, Jay and Brian came from Seattle to visit. Dan and Brian entertained us with some music Sat. night and Sunday we tromped the property trying to convince them they really want to be our neighbors.

Gene felt pretty good yesterday and even drove the tractor out to the back forty to pick up some wood he had left stacked out there from one of his thinning projects. I have run clear out of pine and fir and am burning pure oak, which is hard to start and leaves a ton of ash. I have to admit I gave him some crap because he and a neighbor had cut and split a whole lot of nice firewood last summer and Gene sold a bunch for $50 a cord. I'm sure I can't buy any for that now that he is out of the wood splitting physique! Anyway, I guess I shamed him into bringing in what pine he had out back. I think he had fun.

But today he felt awful all day. I told the doc he was still vomiting and he cannot figure out why. Finally he decided to take him off all meds and see if that helps. So Gene is going cold turkey off the anti-nausea stuff. I wonder if that means the rest of us have to give up margaritas?

TUESDAY, FEBRUARY 13, 2007
11:27 PM

Gene is definitely feeling better! He is not sleeping nearly as much during the day and gets outside for 30 minutes to an hour everyday. Yesterday he hauled a bunch of bags of sawdust the neighbors brought out for bedding in the run in shelters and today he was out raking the driveway. He is wiped out after that much activity but it will help him build back up.

Gene is out of the doghouse about the firewood because our neighbors Del and Jean showed up with a load on Friday. Del said he was used to bailing "Jean" out of trouble, so why not "Gene". Thanks, neighbors!

I had a great horse selling weekend! I sold four on Saturday! Whoo hoo! I hate to see them leave but in the past month I have taken in enough on horse sales to pay the outstanding medical bills through December! Not too shabby! And I have another family trying to get here from Portland to look at ponies, so hopefully one more sale. Then I am pretty much where I want to be unless I can sell one of the Percheron crosses, which would be nice but I also don't mind if I don't. I have had my stallion up for sale, thinking I should not be breeding with my number one ranch hand in poor health and worrying about how hard it has been to get people to come to Goldendale to buy them. But the way they have been flying out the window this week, I am feeling more optimistic about the prospects of selling them. So we'll see. I have cleaned out my pony young stock except for one yearling filly that I have kept hidden because if I get to show this year, I plan on her being my new show buddy.

Tomorrow we go in for Gene's dressing change and will see if they think he is "up" enough to stop our daily IV fluids. It would sure free up some time for getting out to play with my horses! Though Ellie came over today and we did manage to get out for her to ride her Angel pony. And Kalle rode her pony on Sunday. Now if I can just get back to riding my big beauty! I wonder if she remembers me?????

We had a great weekend! Dillon celebrated his seventh birthday at the beach. He had the idea last year that he would like a party at the beach with family and we all had such a great time we convinced him to do it again. We rented the same house, a beautiful four bedroom right on the water. It has big windows and comfy chairs to sit in the warm house with a cup of hot coffee while you watch and hear the surf. You don't even have to go out in the cold. But of course, we all ventured out for daily walks on the beach and enjoyed sitting on the top of the rock sea wall watching high tide crash below us. Gene said the walk back up was tough but he only took a couple of short breathers so I think he did pretty well for a guy with no hair. He felt pretty good all weekend. We ran no IV fluids and he still managed to top 130.

Anyway, all of us except Jill went over on Friday. She worked Friday so joined us on Saturday, then we all stayed till Monday. So a nice weekend! Our beamer got there first and Kalle had to get to the beach first thing. The Risings showed up soon after and waved us in from the deck. Friday night we had take and bake pizza then Rob drew hot tub duty with the kids. After the kids were in bed, Rob and Juli walked on the beach, Gene vegged and I sat in the hot tub with a glass of wine. Not too shabby! Saturday brought more beach walks then we watched Flicka while waiting for Jill to arrive so we could start the party. I tried to decorate the cake like Sponge Bob, but I gotta say, Nana's beautiful cake (Rob's mom always makes the kids beautiful cakes) was sorely missed. But we did have some good belly laughs over pirate sponge bob whose eye slid off the side of his head.

Sunday we loaded up and drove the two miles to Fogarty beach where we watched seals playing in the surf. Sunday night we watched our favorite TV (Desperate Housewives! and Brothers and Sisters!) then Jill and I fell asleep in a rented movie (that no one else even pretended to stay up to watch).

Today we got an early start home to be here in time to load ponies Opie, Manny and Indy up to go to their new homes.

We have a busy week ahead. Jill has an interview at WSU Thursday for vet school. I want to go with her but we are both not sure we are ready to leave Dad to run the show here with school chauffering and all. And the realtor called today to say she has someone interested in a couple of our five acre lots.

But now I am ready for bed! G'night y'all!

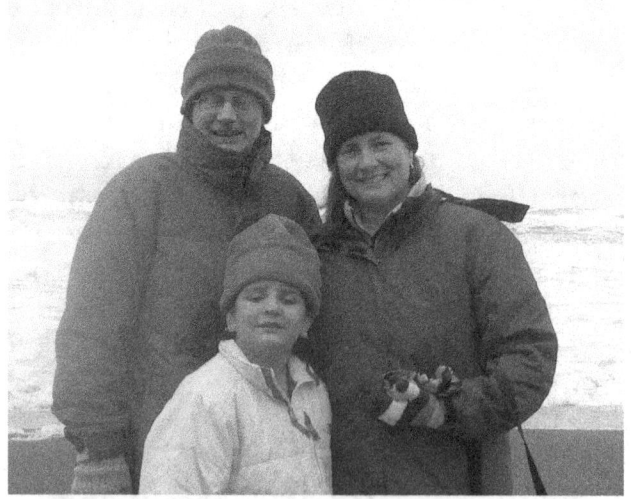

Gene, Kalle and I at the beach

We woke up to snow the past two mornings! Not a lot but enough to look pretty. Today we ventured out to Celilo to get the weekly dressing change done for Gene's PICC line. If he keeps gaining weight without the IV fluids, he may get it out next week! I'm sure he would love to take a shower.

While there, I got the printout from his last HCG (blood tumor marker that indicates germ cell cancer) and it was less than 2! Normal is < 6 and Gene's at the beginning of all this was almost 3000. So this is a GREAT indicator that the chemo has done it's deed. By the way, Lance Armstrong (did I mention we have all been reading his books?) had an HCG level of 109,000 at the beginning of his battle!

Jill had her interview for vet school today. She said she babbled but when she described the questions and answers to us, I thought she did great. So everyone concentrate on getting Jill into vet school! She should hear end of next week. Big times. Though she is a little under-whelmed by Pullman because the hotel did not have Fox so she missed American Idol last night.

I've had a few more calls on horses this week! Only one POA left that I really want to sell though, so now I need some buyers for a couple of big warmbloods!

Gene is getting over his chemo brain. Yesterday he read the whole Lance Armstrong book. Up to now he has not been able to focus long enough to read so this is also big news. Now I'm getting a little nervous that he will catch on to the crazy land deal I talked him into while he was still on the half-there list. I already got caught for some of my creative finances. Oh well. . . When the cat's away. . . I guess that'll make him think twice before he gets sick again!

FRIDAY, MARCH 02, 2007
10:28 AM

GO COUGS!

I guess you might guess from that lead in that Jill did indeed get accepted into the veterinarian program at WSU. So I guess they did not hold either her previous Husky experience or Marianne against her. Marianne is the vet Jill currently works with and she is also a WSU grad. She wrote Jill a great letter of recommendation and when one of the interviewers asked about Marianne (actually remembered her!) Jill thought that must be a good foot in the door. Until she got home and told Marianne who set her straight on that one saying the prof just remembered her because she was always talking in her class.

Oh well, she's in! We had a tense morning Tuesday because Jill missed a call late Monday afternoon and when she called back, the prof had left for the day. Gene and I went to Celilo on Tuesday and had not heard anything from Jill by 10:00 so were getting nervous (she said she would only call us if she got GOOD news). I realized I was as anxious for myself as I was for Jill; I just did not think I could handle seeing her disappointed.

So yippee all the way around. AND Gene got his PICC line out Tuesday so no more artificial appendages preventing him from taking a shower and no more rolling over on pokey things in the night.

He's feeling better all the time. In fact, he just booked a ticket to Albuquerque on March 11 for WORK and has been doing a lot of reading to prepare for the project down there. I can't believe it!

MONDAY, MARCH 12, 2007
9:43 PM

I know everyone is anxious to hear how Gene is doing on his big trip to Albuquerque, working, and all. Well, here is what he says (Fred may tell us it's BS, though. . . Fred???)

Gene said the plane trip yesterday wiped him out so I was a little worried how it would go today. He says he worked from 8:30 till 5:30 except for a nap at lunch while the rest of the crew went out to eat. When I talked to him this evening, he was tired but sounded good; had called for room service and planned a 9:00 bed time (after Prison Break and 24, he thought but guess they weren't on tonight so maybe he even got to bed earlier. Gotta plan the evening around our TV addiction!)

So all in all, sounds like he is doing good. Hope he can maintain it!

Back at the ranch, I dropped the kids off at school then went to Home Depot to buy some drain tubing stuff to run the water from the downspouts away from the barn and also some 2x8's to put around the perimeter so we can dump rock around

93

the outside of the barn without it running under
the wall into the arena which will be filled with
sand. I hauled it all up and parked as close as I
could to the barn without getting stuck in the mud
(road not finished, BAAAD road builder, don't get
me started. . .) then hauled everything by hand the
rest of the way, counting down the trips to pace
myself. I planned on nailing up the boards, but my
hammer and nails had disappeared. I guess the
guy who was working up there hauled them off with
his stuff. Aarrgghh. I guess I will go back
Wednesday to do that. I did get the hole dug and
signpost planted for the road though (Dancing
Mountain Road. Way cool, huh?). Someone has
been up there because the door that had blown off
the barn and was stuck in the mud had been
moved out of the way (thank you) and now one of
the other doors had been unlatched again and was
blowing in the wind (no thank you). Why is it so
hard to get it that these doors need to be latched?
Anyway, no harm done cuz I got it latched before it
blew off this time. The barn is still flooded, which is
depressing, but soon it will all dry out enough we
can get someone in to do the ditching that didn't
get done by the BAAAD road guy in the fall and
haul in the rock, sand, etc to build up around the
barn and inside it. I did discover that my preferred
location for the outside arena is gonna work. It is
low so I was afraid it would be too muddy, but
surprisingly is not as muddy as the higher spot
that would require a lot more site prep. So that was
cool at least. The pond is clear full so it looks nice.
Guess all that water is good for something besides
mud!

MONDAY, MARCH 19 2007
10:04 AM

We picked Gene up at the airport in Portland Saturday evening. We almost didn't recognize him because his head was sporting a brown glow (so much for my grey hair curse) and his beard had grown in. Kalle says he even has eyelashes! In fact, she says her "little bird is growing up into a fine young man."

Sounds like Gene had a good week and came home in great spirits. He even drove home Saturday night! Sunday after church he did some burning and raking, then the Risings came out for Corned Beef and Cabbage and Irish Soda Bread since we got home too late Saturday for a St. Patrick's dinner.

So a good week and a good weekend. Now please hold those prayers for the PET scan on Thursday!

FRIDAY, MARCH 23, 2007
1:18 PM

Well, we're not done yet.

The PET scan shows that some of the lesions are completely gone but the big tumor, though significantly shrunk, still shows up as a hot spot. And one lesion in the liver is gone but the other not.

So now we have to figure out what to do next. Dr. Taylor says we could do another chemo plan, using some different drugs to try to combat the

95

resistant lesions or surgery is also an option at this point since the big tumor has shrunk so much;. Dr. Taylor is worried that it would be a tough recovery though since it would require both thoracic and abdominal surgery to get both spots. Personally, after seeing how tough chemo was on him, I am not so sure surgery recovery would be so bad. At least then you get it over with and can right away get about the business of healing.

But the really GREAT news is that Dr. Taylor is contacting Lance Armstrong's doctor, who is now at OHSU, so he can look at all Gene's records and figure out what to do next. If surgery is the choice, then he can refer us to top surgeons there.

So, while we are so disappointed that the cancer is not all gone, at least they are still looking at options for a cure and that is good news. And Gene is out on the tractor dragging the potholes out of the road.

THURSDAY, MARCH 29, 2007
10:15 PM

hello hello? anybody there? this is Jaimi. I'm wondering why the usual author has gone MIA and if everyone else is speechless or just busy with spring cleaning (minus faithful Al, of course).

Okay, the usual author is probably busy with a lot of things (of which the least is probably trying to decide what the next posting should contain). so instead of being belligerent, I'll help out in keeping people up to date, which is kind of funny since I'm usually the one NOT up to date, being half a world away. Let's chalk it up to being 9 hrs time zones ahead! :)

It's been a bit stressful waiting around to find out when we can get an appointment with Dr. Nichols (Lance Armstrong's doc). In fact, I talked to Mom on the phone Tuesday and we shared exasperation that after 3 working days there was still no progress. I was in the car on the way to a business dinner. When I got home late Tues night, I logged on and searched out Dr. Nichols' e-mail address, then sent a heartfelt plea for attention. When I sent my e-mail, I also downloaded the messages waiting for me: to find that Juli had beaten me to the heartfelt plea-ing and had already gotten a reply from Dr. Nichols! I then called home and talked to Jill - only to find out she had been leaving voice mail messages at Dr. Nichols' office. And then I got Mom on the phone again and learned they had an appointment. Talk about overzealous inundation!

Anyway, if nothing has changed they'll head to the doctor tomorrow. No idea how long it will take to know the next step, but hopefully sooner rather than later. As I'm scheduled to be on ski vacation next week with Kevin, I'll anxiously wait for a phone call Friday night to find out if we drive to Austria or book last minute tickets to Portland because they want to operate. But the good news is: Dad will be seeing an absolute leading specialist in less than 24 hrs! So keep your prayers flowing and fingers crossed!

SATURDAY, MARCH 31, 2007
9:28 AM

Present mood: encouraged but slightly frustrated.

It is such an emotional roller coaster around here, it occurred to me that maybe I should post a mood warning at the top of each entry! Thanks, Jaimi, for filling in while I've been MIA. It has just been another up and down week!

The major downer was that we said good-bye to our good buddy, Chester, our little old TerriPoo. He would have been 16 this year and has been failing quickly since Christmas. We finally made the decision to send him away from pain and cold when he kept falling down and in fact, fell in the pond one night when I put him out to potty. I went out to find him and had to fish him out, shivering and cold. So now he will never be cold or fall down again. Rob, Dillon, Ellie and I buried him on Rob and Juli's property next to our new ranch so he could be next to his life-long friend, Tess, who left us a couple years ago. Ellie and Dillon planted wildflowers on his grave.

This sadness was soon followed by our first foal of the year. I will get her pictures up on the ranch website today. Her name is DMR Dancing in Shadows in honor of the light she brought to our sad week. Her mommy cooperated as usual and gave birth to her in the middle of the afternoon on a sunny day. So she was greeted immediately on arrival by an excited audience of Kalle, Dillon, Ellie and two of our neighbors who I managed to call in time to witness her birth.

I know that is what you all wanted to hear, so I will sign off now.

Just kidding. So the "encouraged, but frustrated" mood of the day follows our visit with Dr. Nichols yesterday. Gene and I drove to Portland for our 1:40 appt and then hurried up and waited about 2 hours to get in. When we did, Dr. Nichols explained that he would need three pieces of information before making the decision for surgery. These are:

1) Current alphafeta protein numbers. This is one of the tumor markers for Germ Cell and he needs to know this because surgery is only indicated if it is still low. He says surgery has not been shown to help in cases where it is high or rising.

2) Another genetic test on the tissue to absolutely classify this as germ cell cancer. The current diagnosis was based on indicative things like high AFP, location, features, etc. in spite of the pathologists classifying the highly disorganized cells that they couldn't specifically identify as lung cancer. Apparently this is a new test that will conclusively end this debate.

3) the surgeons need to review all the scans to determine that they can indeed remove the lesions since the surgery will be tricky at best.

The next bit of information is that if this is NOT operable, Dr. Nichols says it is NOT a bad plan to watch it closely for awhile. He says the PET scans are not 100% and the possibility exists that what we are seeing is actually scar tissue, so it might be wise to watch to see if it actually starts growing again before deciding to do more chemo. So this was actually pretty encouraging since we did

99

not really understand why Dr. Taylor gave "waiting" as one of the options.

So the short story is that we have another appointment a week from Monday, at which time Dr. Nichols should have these 3 pieces of information and be ready to guide us on the next phase of this journey. So the frustrated part is that now we wait again!

WEDNESDAY, APRIL 04, 2007
5:51 PM

Present Mood: discouraged but thankful for Shady in the sunshine.

Yesterday Gene started hurting in his lower abdomen. At first I thought, "Oh crap (yes, I learned that word from Gene), it's the liver lesion growing" but then when he showed me where it hurts, I thought it was too low so started thinking gall stones especially when I read that they sometimes start with pain between the shoulder blades, which he has had for a couple of weeks. Well, we went to see Dr. Taylor today and guess the liver goes way down further than I thought and he is sure that is what is causing the pain. Which is not good news at all.

Also not good news was that his alphafeta protein is up to 168 from 6 a few weeks ago. This probably means they won't do surgery, since that was one of the things Dr. Nichols indicated was decision criteria. But Dr. Taylor said we should keep our appointment for Monday to let Dr. Nichols decide and then if he says go back to chemo we can still do that next week. He also mentioned the possibility of a bone marrow transplant. So Dr. Taylor and Dr. Nichols are discussing the options and we still won't know till Monday, but we are sure discouraged that Gene is feeling bad again. Back to the pain meds.

But I drug him outside to sit in the sun today and he watched Kalle play with the new baby for a couple of hours. Kalle has the baby wearing her jacket in the new pictures. Nothing like a kid, a foal and some sunshine to resurrect a day.

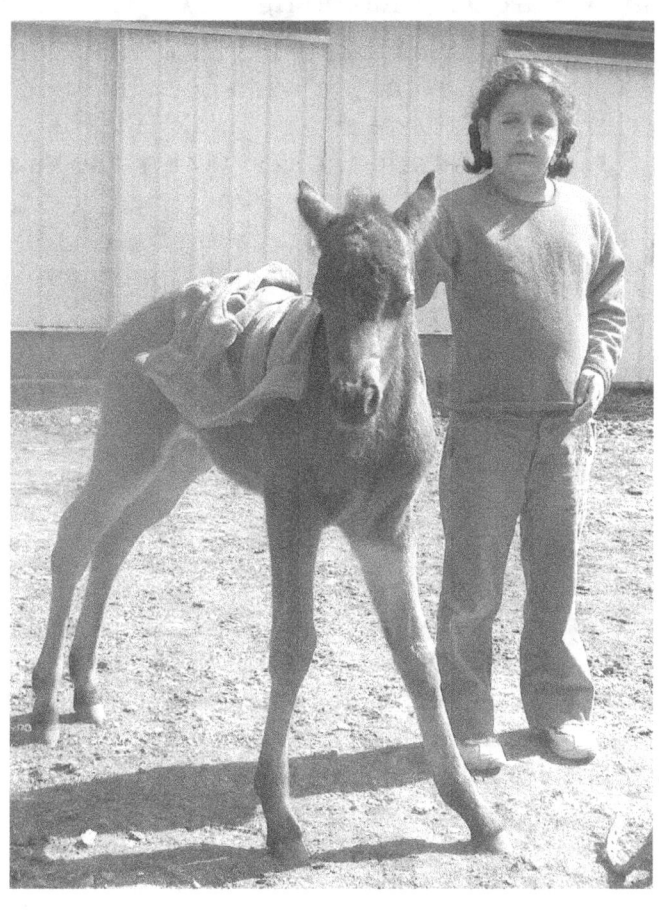

Mood of the day: optimistic

On Monday we made our trek to Portland to see Dr. Nichols. Jillian took off from work and went along and Juli stayed behind to do all the kid shuffling. As we expected, he said that surgery was off the table until the AFP can be brought under control. So he prescribed a new chemo regimen and today we are at Celilo doing Day One of Cycle One.

Gene is receiving two new drugs. One is Gemzar which is said to be especially effective on liver mets and the other is Taxol. He will get chemo on Day 1, Day 8 and if blood count allows it, Day 15 of a cycle. He will have two cycles and then see Dr. Nichols again, but according to the pharmacist here, this is a regimen that is sometimes maintained for a number of cycles. It certainly should be easier on us all than the five long days in a row Gene did before. And the drugs are not expected to have the same puke inducing properties as the last so hopefully we can skip the home IV fluids and bad weight loss!

Dr. Nichols says this is a well established secondary treatment for Gene's type of cancer and some patients have marvelous results with it, so we are praying Gene is one of those "some". And the nurses here talk about the new state of cancer patients which is not cure or failure, but living with cancer, treating it with the best of today's options to keep it under control until something even better comes along. Sort of a hard way to live but a way to live never-the-less!

102

Dr. Nichols also restated how uncommon this lung primary germ cell cancer is and noted that few docs in the country ever treat it, so he was glad that Dr. Taylor brought him in to help prescribe the treatment. We are too!

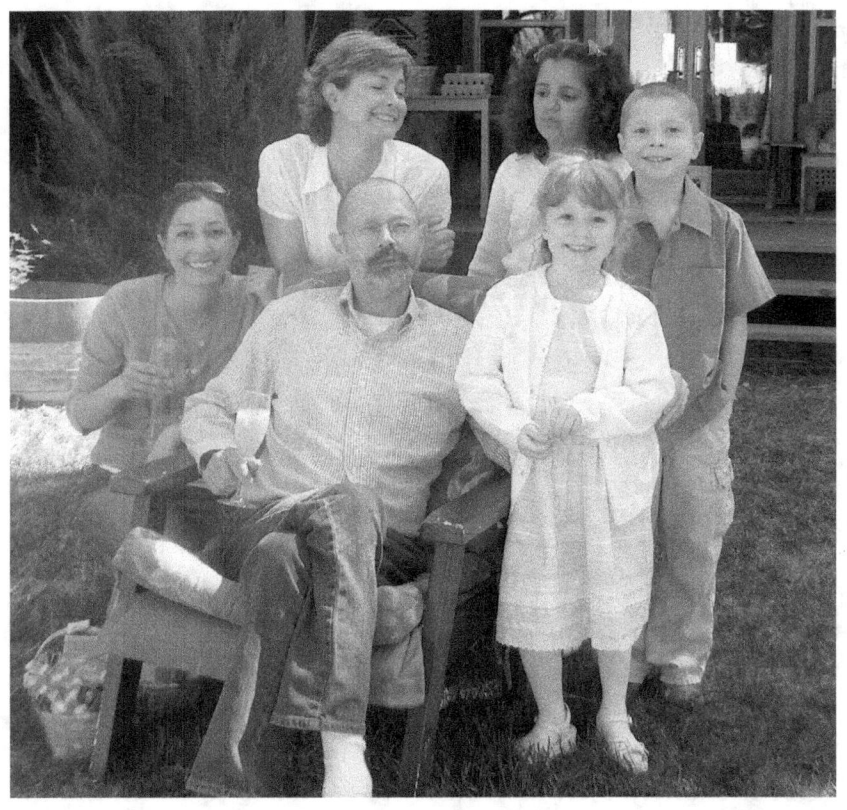

Easter Sunday: Gene with hair, Jill, Juli, Kalle, Dillon, Ellie

FRIDAY, APRIL 13, 2007
1:56 PM

Mood of the day: bummed

Well, I guess we were overly optimistic about this regimen being easier on the tummy. Not. We are back to the puke buckets. And of course therefore having a hard time keeping down the pain meds which he is really needing now. So all in all, not feeling well at all.

Thanks everyone for the encouraging words this week. It is hard to get back into the chemo tolerating frame of mind so we appreciate everyone being there for us. Hopefully in a few treatments the tumors will start to shrink and the pain will go away again.

SATURDAY, APRIL 14, 2007
4:15 PM

Mood of the Day: better!

Yeehaw! He hasn't thrown up for 24 hours! Go Gene Go! We can do this. He is very tired. That is also a side effect of the chemo, plus of course just his body telling him it needs rest to heal. So he is lounging around but definitely feeling better and actually eating so this is major progress. And the pain actually seems a little less horrendous today too.

So good news!

After I wrote the cheery note on Saturday, that night the serious ache to the bone side effect of the taxol hit him big time! But by Monday he was feeling more normal and when we went in on Wednesday he told the doc to hit him with all he had. Thanks to Gene's determination, excellent blood counts, and steady weight, Dr. Taylor decided to give him both the Gemzar and the Taxol again, though a lesser amount of the Taxol this time. We also got a new prescription for Zofran, the really good anti-nausea drug that used to cost $30 a pill but just went generic so is actually affordable and believe it or not--no puke buckets necessary this week! Of course we are still waiting to see if the bone ache starts again tonight, but hopefully with the lesser amount of Taxol, it won't be so bad.

His back is still hurting, though not quite as much, so he is frustrated because he really wants to be out weed-eating and rototilling the garden but just can't do it. Yet. I bet in a couple of weeks he'll be on it!

I finally got out and worked with a couple of horses. I rode Dillon's pony earlier in the week and she did just great. I was not about to put Dillon on her after she had such a long layoff but she did fine, so maybe he will ride her tomorrow. Today I rode Kalle's pony and she also did great so Kalle rode her. Ellie has ridden hers occasionally through all this so no problem there. Ellie was here on Tuesday and got in a ride. I also rode Hope, the big black Percheron today. I just started breaking her last year and have done nothing with her since

105

October so was not sure what she would remember, but she did pretty well for a greeny. She is such a great horse! Gene was sitting out in the sun while I rode and I can imagine him wondering what he was gonna do if she bucked me off!

And baby Shady is already broke to lead and picks up all four feet. So not bad! It's kind of dumb though; all winter when I really could not leave Gene long enough to do much outside I was sad to be missing out on the horses, and now I am having trouble pushing myself to do anything. I guess I am in a lazy rut.

SATURDAY, APRIL 28, 2007
11:41 AM

Since mom is out riding horses, guess I'll have to update the journal! So once again, this is the international update, posted by the author-substitute in Germany. I've been checking daily to see what the latest is myself - after finally getting an update on the phone, decided I'd better let the rest of you in on the news.

Which is a nice job to have, considering the news is quite good! As already mentioned, mom is busy riding horses and enjoying the pre-summer sunshine. Dad is wishing he could do more in the sun, but apparently the taxol is attacking his arthritic knees and it's not real conducive to a lot of movement. BUT: he got his third hit of the new chemo regimen on Wednesday, and all his blood work looked perfect! :) In addition, the extreme back pain he's been suffering from is now gone. So

106

looks like the chemo is doing what it's supposed to do - hurrah!!!

So I went to bed quite happy last night. I mean, what could be better - a Friday evening before a 4-day weekend (in Germany), good news on the home front, and for those of you who don't know, final paperwork indicating that I'm now a Cyrus even in name again! So...wishing you all a great weekend full of sunshine outside and within. And keeping fingers crossed and prayers flowing that the good news continues.

WEDNESDAY, MAY 09, 2007
1:28 PM

We are at Celilo today, starting Day One of Cycle Two. Gene weighed in at 141 (yea!) and his blood looked good. He is still having a lot of pain in his knees, and his hands and feet are numb but other than that feeling pretty good.

We had two fun happenings this week. Steve and Anita dropped in from North Carolina after a wedding at Sunriver. It was great to see them, and Gene was feeling so well that day that we drove down to Maryhill to show them the winery. Fun outing!

Then yesterday we got a big box in the mail from Bud and Cheryl. It contained two of Bud's paintings. One was of the view from our house in Panama and one was of a picture we all loved from a stop in Brugge on our way to Scotland from Germany many eons ago. Both great pictures, but the Panama view one almost made Jill cry.

107

I helped Juli haul her shop to The Dalles last weekend for a scrapbook event. We stayed overnight Friday and got home about midnight Saturday. While we were gone, Gene and Jill worked on Jill's table (she got it to refinish but it has turned out to be a great project for Gene) and also got the early starter plants planted in the garden!

So in spite of chemo and living with cancer, our lives have regained a little more sense of normalcy. Jill is going house-hunting in Pullman this weekend and maybe I will go help!.

TUESDAY, MAY 15, 2007
11:44 AM

Hi everyone, Juli here. Today is my dad's birthday, and unfortunately it is a really tough one... For the past three days he has been in a lot of pain. His lower side/back has been hurting so badly it's been hard for him to breathe. Of course he's too stubborn to let me take him to the hospital (mom went to Pullman to house hunt with Jill Sun/Mon), "for pete's sake, I have my normal doctor visit on Wednesday..." Mom's back and dragging him in today. They will probably do a cat-scan, I will let you know if there is any news... We sure wish we were on a **real** roller coaster for dad's birthday. Please keep us in your prayers, we could really use some long, steady, climbs UP!

Yeah, another roller coaster week. Jill and I had a good time house hunting in Pullman except for worrying about Gene when Juli told us he was miserable Sunday after we left (he played tough in the morning so we would go). As noted, he refused to go to the ER as ordered by his doctor's nurse practitioner when Juli called to tell them about his new pain. So I drug him in Tuesday. We spent his birthday in the ER. They decided the pain was caused by the liver tumor and prescribed him a stronger pain med. Dr. Taylor looked at the CT films on Wednesday when we went in for chemo, and decided it might be good to radiate that tumor now. So he is discussing this with Dr. Steltzer and we will probably be back to the daily drive over for radiation for 5 or 6 weeks. We will find out more about that next week though.

The evening had a better ending, as once again one of our mares came through with a little lightness in the day. Named in honor of Gene's birthday and a very colorful speckled coat, DMR Dancing in Confetti (nicknamed Cupcake) made her appearance about 9:00. I had been checking on the mare every half hour but she didn't act like anything interesting was going on. Then while talking to Jaimi on the phone, I sat on the bed to check the monitor and a baby tumbled into view! She is the tiniest foal we have had; so cute! A black and bay leopard (so white with black and brown spots) with a black face with big white stars and black legs. Shady is getting so big that Cupcake really looks small. With the crazy week, I have not gotten pictures posted but will try to do that soon.

The funny thing about Cupcake's name is that the night she was born, Jill and I were saying we needed to think of a birthday theme name for her. When Kalle saw her the next morning, she said "we should name her Cupcake because she looks like frosting with sprinkles."

Thursday I went with Kalle's class on a trip to the Portland zoo. It was a nice sunny day and we had a great time. Kalle was so excited; she did not sleep much the night before so we slept on the bus ride coming home.

Today Juli and Rob left for a weekend at Salishan; some spa and golf time. Dillon and Ellie are with us. They and Kalle played outside after school until we drug them in for pizza. Tomorrow Jill and I will take them to Shrek 3 so Gene can get some rest. You might imagine that things get pretty exuberant around here when Kalle has her niece and nephew to incite to insanity.

This morning my dad and Barb showed up with a truckload of wood. My dad has been cutting down dead trees at his neighbor's and splitting it onto our old pickup. He and Barb loaded it all up then the three of us unloaded it into the woodshed. It's a lot of work. I tried to convince him to wait until Sunday and make a plea at church for some help but he showed up this evening with another load (after making a trip to town for a new battery for the 73 Chev). My dad is in amazing shape for the downhill side of the 70's. He figures he will have the woodshed completely full by the time he gets it all over here.

So another busy week and not a minute to ride. I think I will send Hope and Grace out for training because I will never get them done at this rate.

Next week will be busy too with a happy event. Jaimi and Kevin fly in next Saturday for a visit. Kevin's goal is to go fishing with Papa, so if we can get the pain under control, Gene is hoping to take him out on the Columbia for some shad fishing. Jaimi ordered some new fishing rods for "the boys" for Gene's birthday. If we can't manage the river trip, we will at least try to catch Kevin a fish in the creek at the corner.

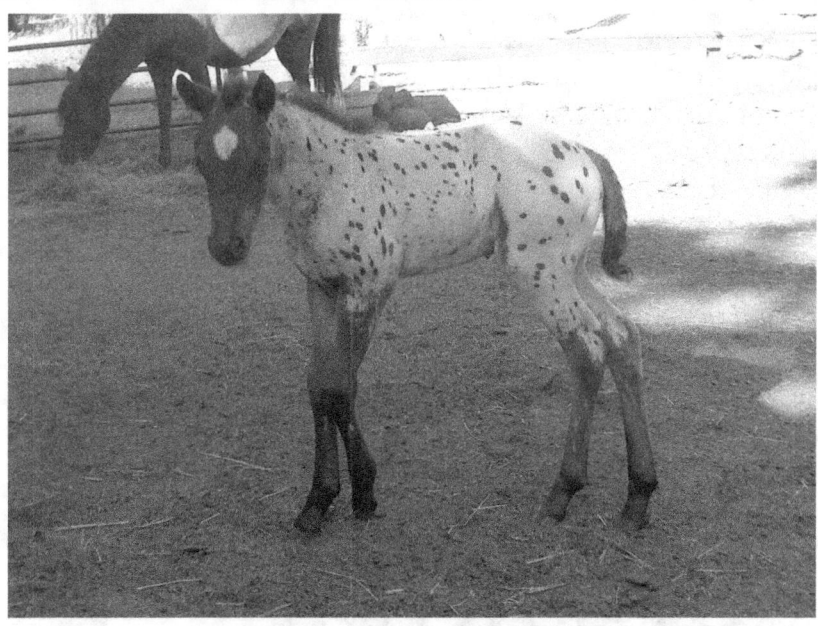

Cupcake: born on Gene's birthday.

TUESDAY, MAY 29, 2007
1:59 PM

Jaimi and Kevin arrived in good form on Saturday. Sunday was kind of windy, so we stayed home and Rob grilled his famous burgers. Kevin and Kalle learned to cast their fishing rods on the lawn, then Kevin spent most of the day fishing in the gold fish pond. Luckily, there was no hook on his line so he didn't snag any of my fish. I told Jaimi he would make a great fisherman: He can sit at the end of his pole all day, happy to catch nothing.

Monday we all loaded up and headed to Horsethief Lake (with hooks) for some "real" fishing. I was the only one who caught anything and it was just a bobber. But it was a beautiful day, a great place for a picnic, and we made it easy with KFC. A good time was had by all.

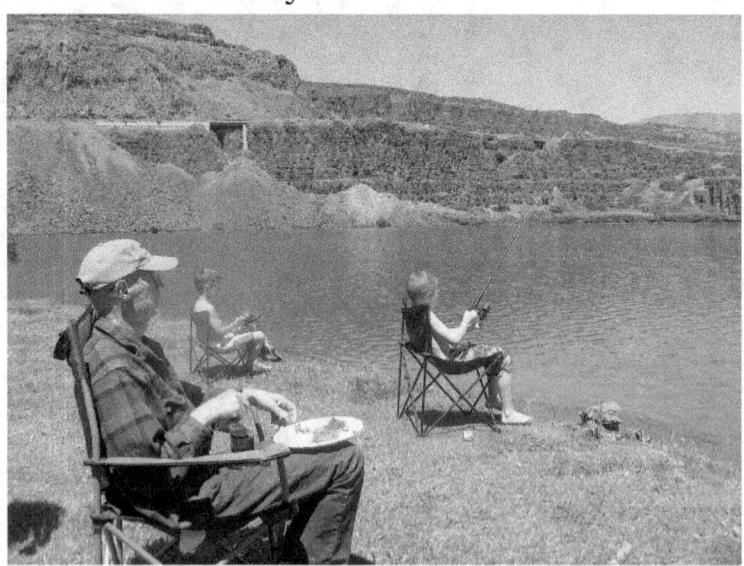

Today he is feeling kind of crummy. Seems like the first of each week following the Gemzar treatment, he has a day of troubled breathing and this is the day he is doing that. But he felt pretty good yesterday and had a good time at the lake, so today is a kick back day and hopefully tomorrow will be better again.

SUNDAY, JUNE 10, 2007
8:53 PM

I am so sorry for the delay in updating the site. I know you are all anxious to hear news but it has been a rough week. In this case, no news did not mean good news.

Gene had his CT scan on Tuesday but we had to wait until Friday to see the doctor (they were all at a national oncology conference earlier in the week, so everyone got backed up). The CT scan did not bring good news. The tumors continue to grow in spite of the chemo. Almost no air is going into Gene's bad lung and the large liver tumor had increased in size and there is at least one new tumor. Dr. Taylor says that in each chemo regimen, the tumors seemed to initially respond to the chemotherapy then very quickly develop a resistance to the drugs and take off again. It is an extremely aggressive cancer, as evidenced in how fast Gene can go from no pain to excruciating pain when the tumors take off again. Dr Taylor felt like further chemo would not be effective against the cancer and just poisons Gene's body. I have emailed some of the images to Dr. Nichols (Lance Armstrong's doc) to see if he concurs but honestly, I am afraid it is a last ditch effort.

I am so sorry for all of us to have to tell you that Dr. Taylor expects the cancer to threaten Gene's life within a few months. He has referred us to a hospice program to get in-home help, primarily to manage pain and help us all deal with what is to come. Gene has continued to have occasional bouts with shortness of breath so we had oxygen delivered on Friday. He also has increasingly unbearable pain in his back. This week they will begin radiation to try to lessen the pain.

You can imagine that we are all devastated. Juli and family, Jill and we have pretty much been in a huddle all weekend. We decided we needed to tell Kalle right away what was going on, for two reasons. One is that she is so perceptive to people's feelings that there is no way she would not intuit that something was going on. Secondly, Kalle has a very hard time dealing with change and surprises. We feel we need to give her as much time as possible to process what is coming.

Several months ago, Kalle asked me if people could die from what her dad had. I told her they could and that that was why he was taking all the yukky medicine and we were all working so hard to help him get well. Last night we called her into the living room and had her sit on my lap. I asked her if she remembered asking this question. She immediately started to cry and asked, "Is my Daddy going to die?" Like I said, very perceptive. We had all managed to put on some pretty stoic faces but as soon as Kalle started to cry, we all joined in. It was the saddest moment of my life, telling this little girl that she was going to lose her daddy.

We cannot understand God's thinking with this. As you know, Gene loves life more than anyone and has done so much good and shared so much love with many people. At this moment, he is very angry to have his life cut short, because, in his words, he still had a lot to do. On the other hand, he sure has packed more into 59 years than just about anyone else I know and he has sure lived a life worthy of celebration.

Jaimi and Kevin were scheduled to come back again the end of July but she has now arranged to return on June 27. We are anxious for her to get home again and feel so bad that she is not here so we can help hold her up in the huddle. It is hard for her at times like this, to be so far away.

Quoting from one of Gene's favorite essays, "The Station[2]" by Robert Hastings: "'Seize the moment' is a good motto, especially when coupled with Psalm 11:24 "This is the day that the Lord has made, let us rejoice and be glad in it". . . So stop pacing the aisles and counting the miles. Instead, climb more mountains, eat more ice creAM go barefoot more often, swim more rivers, watch more sunsets, laugh more, cry less. Life must be lived as we go along. The station will come soon enough."

Gene has surely lived a life full of adventure and love. When we came home on Friday, I asked him if there was anywhere he wanted to go. He said he has been everywhere he really needed to go and now this was the only place he wanted to be.

---

[2]

Used with permission from Southern Illinois University Press, "The Station" from "A Penny's Worth of Minced HAM Another Look at the Great Depression" by Robert J. Hastings, Copyright ©1986 by Southern Illinois University Press.

We hear the whistle blowing but in the meantime, we will all snuggle close ,eat ice cream and Rob's great cooking, watch some sunsets, and listen to the breeze in the pine trees.

Oh man, oh man.
We do what we can
We go through our lives
Whether a woman or a man.
We deal with the ups
And we deal with the downs
We try to make smiles
When we feel more like frowns.
We make friends and grow families
We work through our fears
We just make the best of it
Thru blood, sweat and tears.
Then something comes along
That makes us all sway
We all feel such pain
When God takes away.
A person who could be
The best of us all
From all of us he's the one
God's chosen to call.
We can't understand
God's so much greater than us
We know there's a reason
But he's such a good cuss.
Maybe he was chosen
To show the rest of us the way
Maybe God knew ol' Geno
Would know what to say.
Maybe he knows that wife Judi
Has the strength of ten women

117

Maybe he knows that the kids
Can now go where he's been.
Maybe none of that matters
The way he lived his life
All the friends and the kids
And the wonderful wife.
He would call you a Dork
And you'd laugh and slap backs
Then he'd offer a hand
While calling you a lying sack
But you loved it, you did
Because he did it like no one
He could make a day better
Make your day fun.
I look back myself
At the friends that I've made
And there's no one like him
None at that grade.
He deserved so much better
Yet he got so much more
Because for Gene
Living life was never a chore.
So I salute you dear friend
You're one of the best
Your life here on earth
Was like acing a test.
You touched oh so many
And that will live on.
So don't worry old friend
We'll carry you with us when you're gone.
Love ya
Big Al

Today was a good day. Gene felt a lot better than he has the past few days and even got outside this evening to watch Dillon and I lead Cupcake and help fill the water troughs. We all had a good time tonight eating Rob's great Spaghetti bake and the girls drinking a little too much Dancing Mountain wine.

We went to Celilo today to get the mapping and simulation done to begin radiation tomorrow. Dr. Steltzer plans to radiate the kidney lesion as well as the one causing the back pain because he is afraid it will flare up again and also cause pain. We are happy for him to zap any of those nasty buggers. He plans on doing five treatments so starting tomorrow and finishing next Tuesday.

We met with the hospice nurse, Colleen, and immediately all felt comfortable with her. I met with her first, while Gene was still in radiation. Kalle was with me, and Colleen was a little surprised to find there were no secrets. She acknowledged it would be much easier to work with us than families who are not so open. Kalle told her, "You are my angel of mercy!" Colleen has experience working with children, and will spend some time each week with Kalle, helping prepare her as best we can.

We haven't given up the fight. Today we put together all the necessary material to FedEx out tomorrow to a doctor in New York who uses an enzymatic approach to modifying body chemistry to an environment which is unfriendly to cancer cells. A friend's brother in law was told he had less than

119

six months to live several years ago and now claims he feels healthier than ever in his life on this program. So we will keep you posted on this.

In the meantime, please keep those prayers coming!.

We are so thankful for all the guestbook entries, emails and phone calls. We are so thankful for many loving friends and family. Al's poem really hit close to home to Juli's thinking. When we told her the bad news, she hugged her dad and told him he was the best person she has ever known. She says she does not understand why God would take him; that he already has plenty of good people in heaven and needs more on earth. Rob said maybe God was looking for a good recruiter but then we all agreed that skill is CERTAINLY more needed on earth. In the end, we are still hoping for a grandstand play in the last inning, but we sure have been struggling with the hard questions of "why this?" and "why us?"

We received the following wonderful message for some great friends who we have shared many great times in our lives with:

"The Gene we know never wasted a sunset or anything of beauty or a moment of time, especially if it gave encouragement to a friend, co-worker or family member. The Gene we know has a heart "bigger than the sky" as our grandson says. The Gene we know turns lemons into lemonade. The Gene we know is a magnet to all who cherish friendship. The Gene we know loves his Creator, Savior and Lord. As John Piper says in his book, "Desiring God," "God is most glorified in us when we are most satisfied in Him." Of course, this latest news of your physical condition, Gene, is not what

120

you or any of your family or any of your friends
wanted to hear. We Christians have a very special
blessing of taking the very worst (that which we
would not wish for ourselves or our loved ones) and
turning the circumstances into an opportunity to
glorify Him, something the unsaved and skeptical
may not fully understand. It is about Him, not us.
Not easy, except to the degree you can rest in and
accept that He makes no error or mistake and allows
or causes all things. Not easy, especially when we
work hard to serve Him and honor him and try to
please Him in our marriage, in the raising of our
children and helping those in need. The Gene we
know has done all of these. We don't know why
your situation would be pleasing to Him, but we
trust that He knows, and that one day you and
everyone that loves you will know. That may not
help you feel better about your situation right now,
but we know that one day you will see that is OK,
that as much as your family loves you and your
friends love you, He loves you even more. Not easy
right now, but folks, family and friends who do not
know Him are watching how you have dealt with
and will continue to deal with your situation. They
and all of us want for you what will ease your pain
and give you peace and yes, even joy in "...your time
of trouble." It isn't logical nor fair when viewed
through human eyes. We pray that you two and
each of your children and loved ones will accept His
love, His peace and His joy. To what ever degree
you have served Him, you will stand stronger in
serving Him now. If He is who He says He is, and
who we believe He is, now is the time to crawl up on
His lap and let Him be the daddy you have been to
your children and the grandpa you have been to
your grandchildren. That is where He wants you,

121

resting in Him, so that others will see His love in you.

We love you Gene. We love you Judi. We always will, for we know you as a brother and sister in Christ, and we know that our best times have not yet come."

This message reminded us that God does things in His time, which is very different from our time. We ask how He can take Gene away before we have raised Kalle or before our 75th anniversary (which I fully intended to celebrate at the youthful age of 92) or before Jill finishes vet school or whatever. These things and these times seem very big to us. But to a God who created the world in six days (his days!) they happen in the blink of an eye. Gene says, "but God understands our humanity." which is true, but He also knows that when we join him, we will understand (and experience) God's time and then we will be saying "that wasn't so bad after all."

So even while waiting for the grandstand play, we are seeking peace in the love God and all of you offer us. One of Gene's nurses reminded us that we will all be together again very soon

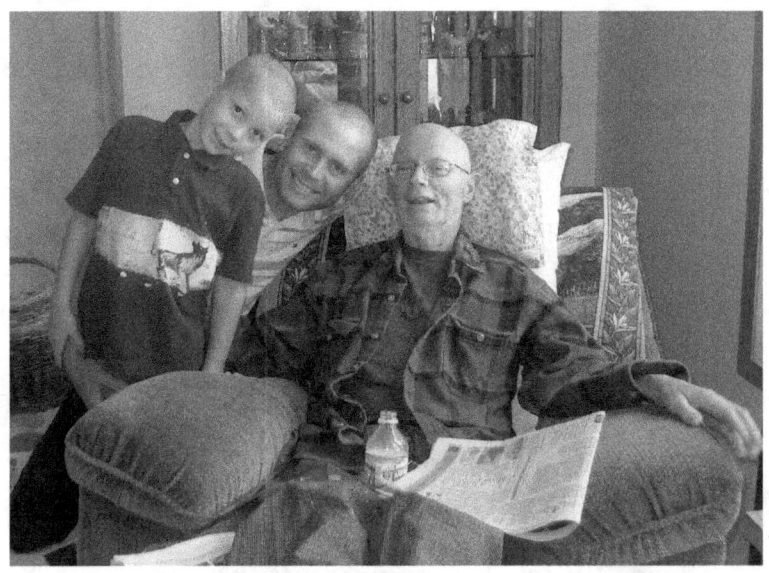

A little empathy goes a long way

SUNDAY, JUNE 24, 2007
12:07 PM

I have been remiss about writing an update. I guess the wind is out of my sails a little bit. But Gene has been nagging me because I did not put "The Station"[3] in it's entirety, so here goes:

"Tucked away in our subconscious is an idyllic vision. We see ourselves on a long trip that spans the continent. We are traveling by train. Out the windows we drink in the passing scene of cars on nearby highways, of children waving at a crossing, of cattle grazing on a distant hillside, of smoke pouring from a power plant, of row upon row

[3] Used with permission from Southern Illinois University Press, "The Station" from "A Penny's Worth of Minced HAM Another Look at the Great Depression" by Robert J. Hastings, Copyright ©1986 by Southern Illinois University Press.

of corn and wheat, of flatlands and valleys, of mountains and rolling hillsides, of city skylines and village halls.

"But upper most in our minds is the final destination. On a certain day at a certain hour we will pull into the station. Bands will be playing and flags waving. Once we get there so many wonderful dreams will come true and the pieces of our lives will fit together like a completed jigsaw puzzle. How restlessly we pace the aisles, damning the minutes for loitering-waiting, waiting, waiting for the station.

"When we reach the station, that will be it!" we cry. "When I'm 18." "When I buy a new 450 SL Mercedes Benz!" "When I put the last kid through college." When I have paid off the mortgage." "When I reach the age of retirement, I shall live happily ever after!"

"Sooner or later we must realize there is no station, no one place to arrive at once and for all. The true joy of life is the trip. The station is only a dream. It constantly outdistances us.

"Relish the moment." is a good motto, especially when coupled with Psalm 118:42. "This is the day which the Lord hath made; we will rejoice and be glad in it." It isn't the burdens of today that drive men mad. It is the regrets over yesterday and the fear of tomorrow. Regret and fear are the twin theives who rob us of today.

"So stop pacing the aisles and counting the miles. Instead, climb more mountains, eat more ice creAM go barefoot more often, swim more rivers, watch more sunsets, laugh more, cry less. Life must be lived as we go along. The station will come soon enough."

124

Okay, so I have fulfilled Gene's request. Meanwhile, back at the ranch, we are still struggling to find the right meds to deal with Gene's pain. So far not much relief. The nurse is bringing out some new meds tomorrow which address more pain receptors than the current ones, so we are hoping that will do the trick. Friday he started taking "superman drugs", a steroid that gives him more energy and he had a good day yesterday, even took care of some mousetraps I have been avoiding (yes, there were mice in them, yuk!) Rob grilled some great burgers last night and Gene even went out to "help". We got a kick out of Dillon telling us how much he likes the new car; we gave the idly sitting Mercedes to them hoping Rob would give it some exercise. Dillon loves the "new" car but when we asked what he liked best about it, he said the trunk. They have never had a car with a trunk before. Then we realized that is also the only car with a trunk we have ever had, too! Funny.

We heard back from Dr. Gonzalez that he does not think his treatment would help Gene. Dr. Sherpa told me Friday that he thinks Sloan Kettering has one of the best cancer centers and they do have docs that have treated Germ Cell tumors (most have not since they are so uncommon!) so we have a message in to them. Should hear back on Tuesday. We also have a call in to a company, recommended highly by some of Gene's sibs, that sells nutraceuticals.

In the meantime, we are just trying to do the best we can with each day that we are given, so please pray for better pain control!

We are at Celilo today for Gene's acupuncture treatment. He finds it very relaxing and hopefully it helps with the pain some. He is now on a new pain med that seems to work better on his back but still gets very miserable before it is time to take it again. During the day we control this with a "breakthrough" drug but he doesn't always wake up in time during the night so mornings are the worst!

We are excited that Jaimi is flying in tonight. Jill is driving to Portland to pick her up. Kevin isn't coming this trip but will be here for the next one on July 26th.

And good news! Paula is bringing dinner tonight! She is a great cook and we are all looking forward to something different than the quicky stuff I have been cooking.

In a couple of days, some of Gene's sibs and families are coming to visit. Sister Leslie will be here with her daughter and family (Kalle is excited to see her favorite "baby" --- now not really a baby anymore though -- Jadzia) then brother Jeff, and Colleen, their daughter, Cheri and family, and son John will be pulling in, the three guys on motorcycles with women and kids pulling a camper popup. On the fourth, their daughter, Heather will fly in from Costa Rica. So big doings are afoot. It will be a little bit of a challenge to keep the house quiet for Gene but everyone is camping on the ranch so should work out okay. We are excited to see them all.

126

I probably won't get back on again for awhile with all the company so everyone have a great fourth.

THURSDAY, JULY 12, 2007
2:27 AM

The family has come and gone and it is quiet around here for a few days until the next wave hits. We had a good time with the gang, though Gene had a few bad days. Still he got up and out for awhile each day and I don't think he ever missed a spot in the audience for the world champion (okay that's a stretch) pickle ball tournament. Juli and Rob were sad to see the gang leave because they don't know where they will ever find such good competition again. It was great fun. And Jill and Heather pretty much mind melded in Cranium giving fits to the competition there.

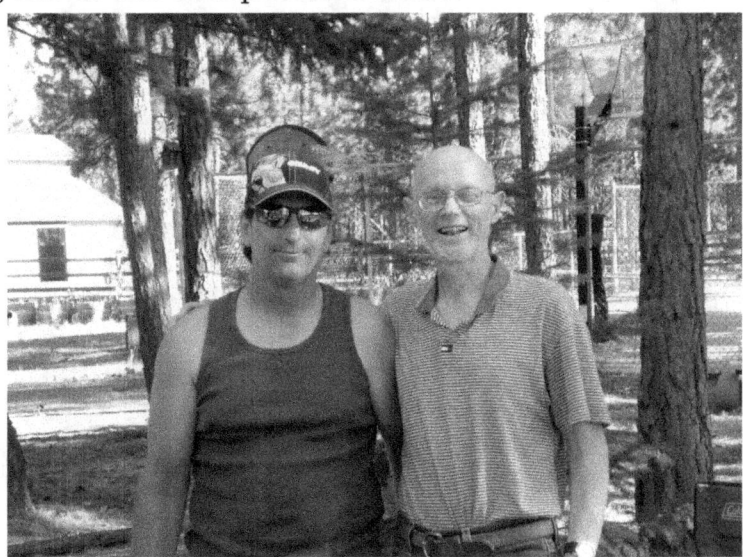

Gene and his little bro, Jeff

127

Kalle survived all the excitement pretty well. Turns out Jadzia is now a threat but she got along very well with Cole. It was good for Kalle to have company. It is hard for her to handle all the excitement, but otherwise it has been kind of a grim summer for her, sitting around watching Dad be sick. We are so thankful to Chuck and Pat for having her over for root beer floats and taking her swimming while they were in town with their grands. It got us started thinking about ways to improve Kalle's summer, so Jill is going to start taking one day a week off to stay with Gene so I can take Kalle on some kind of outing.

Gene has felt better this week. Another couple of med changes and things are under better control. Yesterday he did four loads of laundry, scrubbed out troughs and watered the garden. Today he had acupuncture, so we left Kalle with Juli. She was taking the kids swimming so we came home without her and I got a nice nap in and Juli brought Kalle home later and stayed for dinner.

Jill and Jaimi went house-hunting last week and bought Jill a house in Pullman, so she is now feeling a lot more comfortable about the coming move. She was getting in a bit of a panic about where she was going to live with her large furred family of three dogs and one cat. We are missing Jaimi but she and Kevin will be back again on the 24th.

When Gene tried to get out of bed this morning, his legs would not work. His bladder was full, so I brought him a urinal. He was unable to use it; apparently whatever is affecting his legs is also affecting his bladder. We had to call Hospice and Colleen came out and inserted a catheter.

This was the day we had scheduled a family meeting. I feel like some of Gene's anxiety attacks are caused by his brain whirring around trying to solve all of our little life issues and plan for everything that might happen in the future. Gene still does not believe he is going to die, but he wants to make sure we all know what to do if he does. So he has been making a list of all the things he was worried about, saving it till Jaimi returned so we could all discuss it together. These are the things on his list:

1) Final arrangements: We discussed services. Juli does not want to have one because she doesn't know how she will get through it. Gene told her to suck it up. He wants it on a weekend so work friends can come. And we all agreed we wanted to have it at home where we feel strongest.

2) Jill's situation. We talked about who would go to her white coat ceremony and how he did not want her to change any plans for school because of him. He is so proud of her going off to vet school.

129

3)   Juli and Rob lined up. Juli has to
        move her shop so we talked about
        possible solutions to that. And
        since their house is for sale so that
        they can begin building on their
        property, we talked about their
        moving in here to help me while
        they build. We discussed the issues
        associated with that, most
        especially Kalle's need for private
        time.

4)   Who to see or call. Gene really has
        not wanted visitors and for the most
        part he reiterated that now. But he
        did want to talk to Fred about his
        work. And he agreed that I should
        tell my mom and sister that they
        could come visit. And he said if his
        other brothers wanted to visit that
        would also be okay. He did not
        want his parents to try to make the
        trip because he was too worried
        about their health.

5)   The road and barn at the new
        property. The road up there has
        been an aggravation and stressor for
        two years. The guy we hired and
        paid close to fifty thousand dollars
        never finished the job and did a
        lousy job of what he did do. We
        finally gave up on stressing about it
        and hired someone else to do it. A
        friend of Jaimi's lent us the money
        to do it, since basically we had to
        start over (the new road builder said

it was actually harder to fix what Randy had done than if he had started from scratch, so there was no savings from what we had already paid Randy. But we agreed it is now a problem solved and not to worry about it anymore. We talked about finishing the barn with Rob's help.

6) Hay: We should hire someone to help with it.

7) Clean out office and garage. We all told Gene he was nuts to waste time worrying about stuff like that. He finally agreed and crossed them off the list.

8) Books: He really wanted to make a list of what books I should keep (Terry Brooks) and what ones I could get rid of. I told him this was in the same category as cleaning the garage.

9) Good idea of who gets what down the road. Gene has already given his stamp collection to Dillon and coin collection to Kevin. He kind of wanted to make a list of everything we own and who should get it, but finally agreed that really could wait. He wrote on his notes, "Is this important now vs. leave for the future (then mom has to do by herself). He really was hoping to solve the whole rest of my life for me, I think.

10)   Financial stuff. We agreed to pay off the house mortgage with the life insurance. Hospice has already helped us get Social Security rolling. The girls wanted to spend a lot of time worrying about my financial future, but I finally convinced them I would be all right.

11)   What to do now: we talked about what Gene still needed to do in the time he has. He says he would like to make more of an effort to get outside every day and try to be more physically active. He said it would be cool to take another trip to the beach if he felt better.

It was kind of a strange day. We sat and talked for hours, mostly about practical stuff, but it was comforting to be together, making plans and feeling how much love and support we have for each other. Hopefully this will ease Gene's mind a little and he will feel less anxious for all of us.

SUNDAY, JULY 21, 2007
1:35 PM

Gene has taken a couple of turns for the worse and the day does not seem long enough to get everything done. By Monday he was completely paralyzed from the waist down. He needs help to sit up, lie down, turn over and of course get from bed to wheelchair, wheelchair to recliner and so forth. He went in for an MRI last week and it showed a tumor at the base of his neck that extended into

132

the spinal cord, causing the paralysis. He was treated with radiation for five days, hoping to shrink the tumor away from the spinal cord. It did alleviate numbness in his arms, but did not improve his leg function. There is still some chance for more improvement since the radiation tends to have some delayed effect, but the doctor is not hopeful for a lot of gain, so looks like Gene is in the wheelchair for the duration. He was a pretty good sport about it at first but it is starting to get him down. He just keeps saying he "just wants to walk down the driveway, is that too much to ask?" The upside of the paralysis is that he is not in any significant pain right now.

WEDNESDAY, JULY 25, 2007
4:39 PM

We are thankful that my mom and sister Norma were here last week, especially to help get Gene in and out of the car to go to treatments. Thankfully he married a big cowgirl that can heave him around, but aiming him into the car door really requires an extra person. I can do it by myself but it is a little scary. I park the wheelchair alongside the car, have Gene put his arms around my neck, I put my arms around his waist and my right leg between his two legs, then lift him up and pivot him around. Next comes the tricky part. I have to somehow push his bum back into the car enough so that when I let him down, he will be on the car seat enough for me to then push him on in. One time I missed and he almost ended up on the ground. We both had some pretty wide eyes before I got him up and in. I had the most awful helpless

133

feeling so I can imagine how he felt, unable to do anything to save the situation.

Jaimi and Kevin got back yesterday so we are huddling in the "family bed" with lattes half the day. Colleen, our hospice nurse, offered us a hospital bed, which she said would make it easier for turning, bathing, etc but noted that it would be harder to get our whole family into. She has been around enough to know that we all lay around in the bed talking in the mornings and evenings. My dad has been coming over regularly to help Gene with his "God questions" and he sits in the wheelchair next to the bed while we all lay around in it.

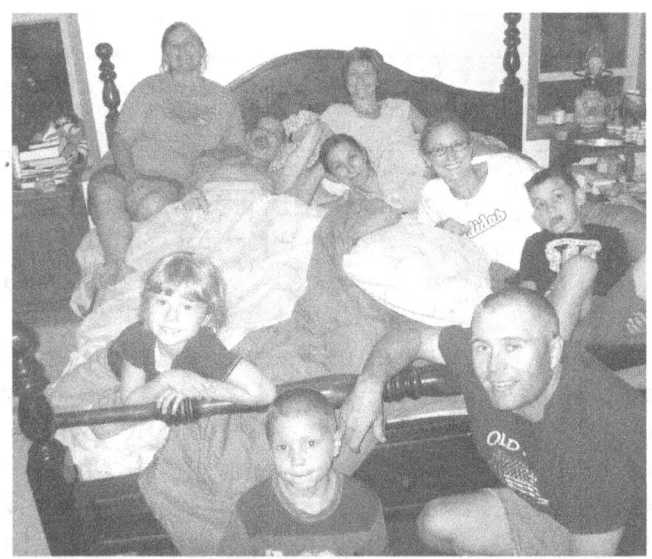

We could have gotten one more in but someone had to take the picture!

Mom commented that she has been around sick people who become very cranky. We all marvel that Gene continues to worry about the people around him. He asked Mom and Norma several times a day if they were doing okay. It's hard to imagine being so sick and worrying if everyone else is okay. Of course, I believe that has been the cause of some of his anxiety attacks. He is so worried about what will happen to the rest of us, especially Kalle, when he is not here to take care of us.

Gene has been reluctant to have many visitors; he feels like he needs to entertain them and wears himself out. In fact, initially he resisted Mom and Norma's visit, but finally acknowledged that they needed to be here for me. After all that, he has really enjoyed having them, even asking them to extend their visit. He has had several great conversations with both of them, most notably telling my mom that he "sure had fun being married to her daughter for 37 years." Mom will treasure this always. Who could ask for more for a daughter than that her husband love her his whole life?

The wheelchair has turned out to be major entertainment for the rest of the family. We can all pop wheelies in it. The kids take turns racing around the house in it. When Cathleen, the hospice chaplain was here, she noted the high activity level with the wheelchair and said, "We could bring another one. We have lots of wheelchairs."

Thursday evening Jill's boss is taking the whole vet clinic and as many of our family as can make it to Romuls in The Dalles for Jill's going away dinner. We are drawing straws here to see who goes. Then the first week in August, Jill should close on her house and we will have some moving trips over. Her white coat ceremony is August 17th (also her birthday) and some of us (including Jaimi flying in from Germany) will make it to that. So big happy events also happening in the middle of all the pain.

And of course our little ones continue to fill our hearts with joy. Gene told Dillon he was going to give him the stamp collection and Dillon asked if he could look at it with him so he could keep that as a memory. A few weeks ago Dillon had a bad day when he was sad and crying. He told Juli he was sad about papa cuz he prays every night for a miracle and why can't he get a miracle? Last week, riding in the car, he suddenly said excitedly, "Mama, I know!" Juli had no clue what he was so excited about, but he went on, "I know why Papa is going to heaven so soon. It's cuz Papa already has so much love in his heart he's ready to go to heaven. He doesn't have to stay here till he's old." It's the best explanation we've heard so far so we are clinging to that.

SATURDAY, JULY 28, 2007
2:37 PM

Yesterday we decided to get beyond the "getting down" over the paralysis issue. I told Gene we could either get up every morning with probably unrealistic expectations of it being better and thereby set ourselves up to be disappointed every morning or we could just accept the assumption that at this point in this journey, things probably are not going to get better and just get on with making each day the best it can be. So we set goals for yesterday by which we would judge it to be a good day. Our goals were to get outside for awhile, hold hands, take a bath and exercise those poor little legs. We achieved all those goals and it was indeed a good day.

I took Gene outside to water the garden while I fed horses yesterday afternoon. He was sitting in the wheelchair watering when Jaimi came home so he had her wheel him over to water the aspen tree grove. They sat there together, talking and watering, then I guess Gene decided to wheel himself back up the incline to the driveway. This turned out to not be such a good plan, as he flipped the chair over backwards and when I came running to Jaimi's yell for help, he was laying on his back in the chair with his feet sticking up in the air. Fortunately he was not hurt, but looks like we need to put in a request for a ranch tested four wheel drive wheelchair!

Today Rob and Juli are coming to grill steaks for dinner so it will be pretty easy to make this a good day!

Our neighbor, Jean, mentioned in the guestbook about visiting with Gene while they helped with hay. I forgot to mention that last week we had about 12 tons of hay delivered and dumped in the driveway. The first four tons Norma, Jill, Breanna and I stacked in the barn. It was the day Norma and Mom arrived and I got the giggles because they arrived on Monday instead of Tuesday only because Norma did not get called out for work Sunday night. I told her I bet she was wishing she HAD gotten called out! The rest of the hay was moved and stacked thanks to efforts from our neighbors Del and Jean, Mark and his brother's family (visiting from S. Carolina), Chuck and Pat, and Ron. Thanks all!

Now I only have thirty tons to go!

137

Yesterday friends of ours visited from Seattle. Gene did not think he would feel like company, so we left him in bed. We visited while he slept most of the morning, but when he woke up for lunch, he said he would like to see them. So Dan and Ann sat in the wheelchairs (oh yes, we have two now!) while family sat on the bed, and we talked. Mostly we talked about kids and work and all that small stuff. Suddenly, out of the blue, Gene asked, "Dan, what is the first thing you will say to God when you get to Heaven?" This was momentarily met by stunned silence as we all processed this question. Finally I laughed and told them that Gene was the only person I know who has written a To Do list for when he gets to Heaven. This is Gene's list:

1. Look for people I know
2. Ask for the orientation Angel
3. See what God looks like
4. Watch and feel his arms around me and ask a bunch of questions
5. Do a 360 to see the panorama of heaven
6. Ask about Kalle[4]
7. Find the phone to call home

The next day, Dan sent an email saying, " *I am sending Gene a hand stitched journal - hopefully Gene can capture some of his thoughts . . . When he asked the question 'What is the first question you would ask God' it really threw me for a loop (for a*

---

[4] Kalle, who we adopted in Panama in 1998, has brain damage caused by head trauma when she was a baby.

number of reasons). But wow, what an ice-breaker. Gene's never had trouble with that. I liked the question brain storming session. Even thought it might make for a good book - Questions to ask God. I have a ton of them. But I'm pretty sure, if there is an afterlife, and I somehow end up on the right end of it I will need a tour guide. Me thinks Gene will be filling that role."

By this time, Gene could not write legibly, so Jaimi made the first entry in the journal:

"Our family is special in the way that for each one of us, our very best friends are other members of our family. We've traveled throughout the world, met many people and come to feel at home in lots of places, but when we think of friends and comfort, we most often turn inward.

"We are now at a time that we cherish this bond and this friendship, and prepare for a momentous good-bye. The first really important one for several of us. And it is in preparation of this good-bye that a friend of the family presented us with this beautiful journal. Within its pages, we will capture some of the thoughts, prayers, feelings and important lists that have marked the progression of Dad's exit—his preparation for closure of this life and entry into the next. And as much as we mourn and are saddened by the impending good-bye, we are joyful that it will be followed, in moments or lifetimes" by meeting again.

Thankful for the life, experiences, and love and support of this unique family, Jaimi"

Just a quick update because I know people are anxious for news. Not much time; since Gene is paralyzed he needs a lot of help so I am pretty busy. But he is stable at the moment, sleeping quite a bit but talkative when he is awake, and his pain is well controlled. I loaded him up yesterday because we needed groceries so he got a ride into town, then we drove up to the property to see how the road is coming. We now have the right guy working on it and it is beautiful. Sadly, we learned last week that HE just found out he has cancer so please add Jim to your prayer lists.

We had other terrible news this weekend. My dad and his wife drove to So. CA last week for a wedding and my dad suffered respiratory failure Friday night. He has asthma and the pollution may have been too much for him. He was without air awhile and suffered cardiac arrest. Some other hotel patrons performed CPR till the paramedics got there who defibrillated him a number of times and got him to the hospital. He has been there in a coma and on a respirator since then. We are shocked and devastated. It would be a hard deal anytime but you can imagine the timing of this almost seems personal. I, of course, want to fly down and be with him while at the same time want and need to be here with Gene. Fortunately my sister, Sondra, and her husband drove from Phoenix to California Friday night and have been there since early Sat morning. Gene is climbing the bedrails wanting to get up cured to take care of Granddad (as he calls him) and me. He says, "Now

I really have to get well." My dad is a Christian and looks forward to his trip to heaven but this is not a good time for me to let him go. It is hard to believe he could have single handedly cut, split, loaded, hauled and stacked enough firewood to fill my 10x16 wood shed earlier this summer and then have this happen. A few days ago, Dad stopped in to see Gene before they left for California. He said good-bye not knowing if Gene would be here when he came back, but it never occurred to any of us that Dad would not come back.

The hospice nurse was here today. Gene complained to her that he was sleeping a lot and just could not stay alert. She said, "That is part of the process." Gene said, "Does that mean you think I am going to die?" She smiled at him and said, "I'm saying it's part of the process." Gene is still holding on to hope for that miracle.

Colleen and I talked about my dad and how I was so torn about going down there vs. leaving Gene. She pointed out that Gene has been very stable and pretty much pain free for the past couple of weeks, has been eating well, etc. so she thought it would be a good idea for me to go to say good-bye to my dad

After she left, Gene asked me again when Jill's white coat ceremony is. I told him on Friday. He said, "Oh! That soon. I don't know if I'll be ready yet."

Other but better news is that Juli and Rob helped Jill move into her house in Pullman this weekend. Jill is thrilled with her house but surprised how fast she is filling it up with all the stuff she forgot she had in storage while she has lived here the past two years. Her white coat ceremony is Friday and the plan is for Juli and Rob to stay here with Gene while I run over for that and Jill's birthday dinner (30 big years!) but of course we make every decision a day at a time.

I got in trouble with the hay report because I forgot the load that Juli, Rob and Jill stacked! We still haven't started on the 30 tons at the other barn but will need to do that before the rain starts.

So, dull and slow around here as you can see.

WEDNESDAY, AUGUST 15, 2007
8:36 PM

Juli and Rob got home from Pullman Monday night, Juli stayed over with me and I left at 3 am to catch a plane to southern CA. I got to my Dad's side about 10:00, spent about 5 hours there then flew home to arrive back at Gene's side at 10:00 pm. I am so glad I went.

Juli and Rob had a great day with Gene. Rob and Gene had a heart to heart talk which I learned of when I found notes in Rob's handwriting regarding Gene's worries about me and my inability to ask for help. And Colleen had a trapeze for Gene's hospital bed delivered. Gene is sporting some pretty good biceps again because he has been building up his arms lifting dumbbells while sitting in his chair. So Colleen thought it would be good if he had a way to move himself around in bed better. Well, Juli says he had a blast swinging from the trapeze like a monkey all day.

They did an EEG on my dad Monday and another on Tuesday. The hospital and my sister, etc. called here this morning to tell me that Dad's

142

renal function had worsened to where his kidneys were not functioning at all. He had a fever, they have been fighting pneumonia, and the second EEG showed degradation from the first, which indicated only about 2 percent of his brain was functioning. So we made the hard decision to turn off the ventilator. He has continued to breathe on his own, but body systems are failing, so barring a miracle it is only a matter of time till he leaves us. I personally think he is waiting for Gene, so they can walk into God's presence together. I told Gene that and he said he would like that. He and my dad have become pretty close, especially in the past few months. They were golf buddies last year, but this year they have become Bible buddies.

As if all that weren't enough, Kalle discovered her little finch (bird) dead this morning. She cried loud wrenching sobs for about an hour, raving about how she loved the bird so much and had so much fun with it and had so many plans for it. We all knew she was not really talking about the bird but it sure was the last straw for a little girl living on an emotional roller coaster. Juli saved the day; she came out to get Kalle and took her to buy a new bird. When they got home, we got the new bird (named Beep Beep Stripes --zebra finch) settled, then had a funeral for the old one (Peep aka Beep). I sang a lovely song: "Once there was a little bird whose name was beep, beep, beep and Kalle loved that little bird whose name was beep, beep, beep. He used to beep and sing all day but now he's gone to Heaven today. Kalle loves that little bird whose name was beep, beep, beep." Okay but it was spur of the moment so give me a break. Then we all sang This Little Light of Mine and Kalle did a eulogy hoping Beep is in a happy place, Dillon did a prayer and Juli managed to keep mostly a straight face, though she and I both lost it a little during my beep beep beep song.

Gene had a rough day today; it was good I went to CA yesterday. The tumor in his back seems to be growing again and is causing great pain so we increased the pain meds and he slept most of the day.

We are all exhausted and praying for no more testing of our mettle.

THURSDAY, AUGUST 16, 2007
7:48 PM

Gene lost his hard fought battle this morning. He never gave up hope for that miracle and never stopped wanting to be here for his family in spite of all the pain and illness. But in the end his spirit could not conquer the terrible beast. At one point in the battle, when he acknowledged he MIGHT not win, he told me he would feel like he was letting everyone down and that he should not give up. I asked him if, when he was running in college, he thought he "gave up" when he came in second (i.e. didn't win the battle). Fighting to the end is a win in my book, even if you don't win the race.

Thank you all, dear friends and relatives, for all your support and encouragement through this hard journey. We know you will all miss him so much, as we already do.

My Dad passed away early this morning.

Since my dad continued to live without the life support, my sister Sondra and her husband had made arrangements to have Dad moved by ambulance to their home in Phoenix should he have lived until Monday. They were there with Dad throughout the week and were committed to caring for him as long as necessary. It was such a gift to me to know they were loving and caring for him while we were dealing with our own heartbreak and challenges here.

We are in shock over so unexpectedly losing my dad but also shocked over losing Gene. Juli and I both felt like we knew his illness was claiming his life but after it did, we can't quite believe it really happened. It has been a hard week.

In the past few weeks, Gene has sort of resigned himself to that miracle not happening. He has asked that if it is God's will to take him, what is he waiting for. Enough with the suffering. I read him a quote from "The Reluctant Messiah" that says if you are still living, your mission is not complete. Gene wondered what sort of mission he could be expected to accomplish in the shape he is in. But now I believe his mission was to be here when I got the news about my Dad. We held each other and cried together. Gene asked me to say a prayer for Granddad, which I started but was unable to finish, so Gene took over for me.

Gene used to be the typical reserved Lutheran dad. He always appointed one of the kids to say the blessing and while his faith was obvious in the way he lived and treated people, he never really vocalized it. In the past months he has become a lot closer to God, has studied the Bible, asked tough questions of the hospice chaplain and his "model Christian" Bud, and prays with me each night. We have struggled together to understand this whole ordeal and have come to the conclusion that God did not do this but he gives us courage and strength to get through it somehow. We have heard from people who say that if you claim healing from God and have faith you will be healed. We have heard from people who believe in miracles and tell stories of miracles, and we have asked for our own miracle. If anyone ever asked harder, believed more, or deserved more a miracle, it is Gene. I no longer believe in miracles because I can't believe in a God who would arbitrarily grant miracles to some and withhold miracles from others. Some people claim that if you are not healed, it is because your faith is not strong enough. Baloney. Obviously the death rate on earth is 100%.

The best book I have read during this time of searching is, "Why Bad Things Happen to Good People." The conclusion of this book is that there is contradiction in the beliefs that 1) God is all powerful, 2) God is loving and 3) God is Just. We have sure seen the contradiction because if God is loving and just AND all powerful, Gene would surely have received his miracle. God IS very powerful: he created the heavens and the earth. But he created the earth according to a design of natural laws and free choice which in a way was a forfeit of his ability or inclination to be all-powerful on earth. He wouldn't create such a world and

146

then micro-manage it, violating the very laws he created.

Okay, it is not really true that I don't believe in miracles. Life is a miracle. Creation is a miracle. Springtime is a miracle.

But I don't believe we necessarily get what we pray for or even what we deserve on earth. Surely I did not deserve to lose my husband and my dad in the same week, or my children their father and grandfather. And surely Gene deserved that long and productive life he so fervently prayed for, deserved to see Kalle grow up and Jill graduate from vet school and to fish with his grandkids.

Gene came to the point where he said he no longer knew what to pray for, so we began to say the Lord's Prayer together. For the first time in my life, the phrase, "Thy will be done on earth as it is in Heaven." held new meaning to me. It says to me that God's will IS done in Heaven and we look forward to the time when it will also be done on earth. But right now, at this time on this earth, maybe it isn't.

Yesterday (Friday) Rob, Juli, Dillon, Ellie, Kalle and I drove to Pullman to be with Jill for her white coat ceremony. When I called her Thursday about her dad, she wanted to come home but we said we would go to her instead. Jaimi flew in to Pullman late Thursday night so was there too. Thankfully, Jill's wonderful friends Marianne and Tracy drove over to be with Jill on Thursday so she did not have to be alone in a town of strangers on such a hard day. On Friday, my mom and sister Norma joined the crowd, so Jill had a large cheering section at the white coat ceremony and her birthday dinner afterwards. Mom and Norma came home with us today, where my brother George joined us from Denver. Thinking back on Gene's comment Monday about not being ready by then, referring to Jill's white coat ceremony, I realize that I misunderstood what he was saying. At the time, I thought he meant he would not be well enough to go by then and my reaction was kind of "Duh!" I told him we were not planning to go, that Juli, Rob and Jaimi would be there for her and that Granny and Norma were also hoping to go, so he should not worry about it. Now I think he was planning on all the rest of us going but on Monday was not sure he would be ready to leave us in time. I guess he was. He definitely wanted everyone to be there for Jill. He was so proud of her making this big step.

Many have asked about services and remembrances for Gene. The girls and I decided this morning to delay Gene's memorial service in case I needed to go south again because of my dad. Turns out there will not be a need (or opportunity) for that but we will stick with the plan and hold a memorial service for Gene on the weekend after Labor Day, probably on Saturday the 8th. I will post the details soon. As for remembrances, when we were working on building the new church and planning landscaping (a job we have not followed through on during Gene's illness) we made a plan for a future outdoor worship area. Now I want to implement that plan as a memorial to my Dad and Gene. Anyone wanting to participate can send memorial gifts to Christ the King Lutheran Church in Goldendale. Or if you have been particularly thankful for the Caring Bridge site, you could make contributions here for that.

MONDAY, AUGUST 20, 2007
11:14 PM

We will hold the celebration of Gene's life on Saturday, September 8th at 4:00 pm. In keeping with Gene's casual approach to life and love of home and outdoors, it will be held in our backyard. It will be a "bring your own lawn chair" casual type service and dress accordingly casual. We will also share one of his favorite eating opportunities with a potluck supper.

Jaimi will fly in from Germany to Portland about noon so we are hoping she doesn't encounter any delays!

WEDNESDAY, AUGUST 22, 2007

From the Goldendale Sentinel:

Gene Raymond Cyrus (59) was born in Minneapolis, MN on May 15, 1948 to Gordon Arthur Cyrus and Marian Ruth Perry Cyrus. Gene was raised in an exuberant family of 6 siblings (one girl and five energetic boys) and he carried that exuberance over into all aspects of life and into his own family. Gene, who never met a stranger, was commonly known as "Hi, I'm Gene," one of the most-used phrases in his life through his outgoing approach to meeting new friends all around the world. He graduated from Ishpeming High School in Michigan, attended Itasca Junior College where he is still renowned for his athletic prowess in cross-country and track, and then continued on to finish his studies at the University of Minnesota where he graduated Magna cum Laude in Business Administration. In 1969 while visiting his parents, who then lived in Rifle, CO, he noticed a beautiful appaloosa ridden by the neighbor girl. He asked his brother who the girl was and to

149

his brothers question of "why, do you want to meet her?" he retorted with "no, I want to ride her horse!" A year later, he married that girl next door, Judith Lynn Johnson, and began their inspiring life of 37 years together. They were joined in their life adventure by their three daughters, Juli Dawn Rising of Goldendale, WA, Jaimi Kristen Cyrus of Boeblingen, Germany, and Jillian Lindsay Cyrus of Pullman, WA.

Gene began his career in Human Resources for the U.S. Forest Service in Albuquerque, NM. He devoted the next 28 years to Human Resources management, working for the Forest Service and the Department of the Army. His career, combined with the family's natural penchant for adventure and love of life, brought them to many stations in the western part of the US, Germany, and Panama. The Cyrus outlook embraces broad life experiences, leading them to many travels and shared adventures. The family's enthusiasm and closeness stimulated a desire to share their lives further, and in 1995 they adopted a sibling group of six (Michael, Crystal, Wesley, Joseph, Doloras, and Breanna) and in 1998 a Panamian infant, Kalle Bethania.

In addition to traveling, Gene loved fishing and hunting, planting trees, gardening, fighting forest fires (professionally for the forest service and managing his own while landscaping), downhill skiing, coaching his daughters' sports activities, and executing all his wife's ambitious plans.

Both professionally and privately, Gene's interactions with others were unique in that people always walked away feeling good – about themselves and about life. An eternal optimist, he was known for his loyalty, good humor, witty puns, generosity and above all, his magnetic charisma.

Tragically, on August 16, he lost his fierce battle with germ cell cancer, despite his active and healthy lifestyle and positive outlook. He is survived by:

His parents, wife and children
His sister, Leslie Kaye and his brothers Larry, Dennis, Jeff and Kim
Son in law and fellow grillmaster Rob Rising
Grandchildren Dillon, Ellie, and Kevin
Hundreds of close friends and colleagues around the world

WEDNESDAY, SEPTEMBER 5, 2007

I spend my nights searching the house for signs of Gene—notes, keepsakes, something that ties him to the earth and me, or lifts me to heaven to him. During one of these nightly tear apart the house searching episodes, I found an unused journal on the bookshelf next to some books written by a Hawaiian friend of my dad. The title on the front of the journal is "New Beginnings." Maybe that's for me although it feels so much like an ending. I guess this is stupid after 38 years, but I did not think I would miss him this much. I thought I would be okay, that it might even be a relief not to see him suffering and not to be so tied down. I was so wrong. I miss him so much. And I miss who I was with him. I forgot the shy, insecure girl I was when I met him, that I used his outgoing-ness and confidence to carry me along.

I thought I would find comfort in the horses but I find I really don't even care about them. I slug around feeding, hardly seeing them and certainly offering and receiving no comfort. How can the loss of Gene change this in me? The horses were always my passion—which he indulged me in but never really shared. So why does his not being here take away this passion?

151

And our house! It is so beautiful and peaceful here. It offered me so much comfort when Gene was sick; I would sit by his bed and look out the windows at the aspen trees we planted by the playground, watching the leaves quivering in the breeze, bright with spots of sun and shadows. But now this place that we put our hearts and souls into feels like an albatross. I want to run away from it.

I guess this was an especially bad day because Saturday is the memorial service, which I guess sort of makes this all reality and not just a bad dream I will wake up from. And Sondra and Don will arrive tonight so tomorrow we will be taking care of Dad's things.

THURSDAY, SEPTEMBER 6, 2007

Today was a better day. It was really good to see Sondra and Don and mostly we were so busy that I just got through it. Tonight Bud and Cheryl arrived and we all had dinner together. We looked at the photo album Juli made for Gene for Father's Day and just talked a lot about him. It was good. And the bottle of wine didn't hurt either.

WEDNESDAY, SEPTEMBER 12, 2007 10:06 AM

Saturday was a beautiful, Gene kind of day. It was sunny, the grass was green, the mountain white capped, horses leaned through the fence to munch on the grass, and we were surrounded by friends and family. Dan, Doug, and Rich provided beautiful music, and Bud, Fred, Steve, Denise and Sandra moving tributes. And we had lots of great food and beautiful flowers.

Thank you all who shared in that day and in this entire journey. It has been hard, but we have felt your gifts of love, support and friendship all along the way.

It was really a pretty uplifting day. As I noted to many, it would have been a great get-together other than the reason for it. And now that all the guests are gone and the quiet gathers around, I begin to really have to come to grips with that reason. This is the hard part. The house is quiet and I don't know which way to turn. I want to stay in bed with the covers over my head. But then there is Kalle and I have to keep going for her. But I am so tired.

Children's Message
from Baba in Memory of Papa

"Hey guys, there are a lot of people here today, aren't there? Why do you think so many people came to see us today? Well, they are here because they want to remember Papa Gene with us. We are all here to talk about him and about how much he meant to each one of us. There will be lots of stories. Some will make us laugh and some might make us cry.

But I want to talk to you about how Papa Gene will always be with us.

Who knows what this stick is?

Right, it was Papa Gene's walking stick. It is a special kind of stick that he got when we lived in Germany. It was actually made by two tree

153

branches that grew together for awhile, twisting together. The old German guy who made this into a walking stick, took the little branch away but you can still see its imprint where it grew into the big branch.

An imprint is a mark on something that reminds us of something else.

A fossil is an imprint.

I can make an imprint by pressing this silver dollar into this clay. See, you can actually see something like a picture of the coin when I pull it away from the clay.

That's an imprint.

Well, all these people are here today because Papa made some kind of an imprint on each one of them. And he especially made an imprint on each one of you. Who can think of an imprint he made on you? [Kalle says, "He taught me to burp" and mom says "You also have his sense of humor.]. Dillon is like Papa in the way he thinks hard about things. Ellie is like Papa when she is cheerful.

So in a way, Papa will always be here where we can see him when we look for his imprint on the people he loved.

Papa collected a lot of these silver dollars, so I will give each of you one of them. Keep it on your table by your bed, and when you are missing Papa, think about imprints and know that Papa is still here because you have his imprint on you."

EULOGY FOR GENE CYRUS
May 15, 1947, 1920 – August 16, 2007
By George Inslee

*Before I begin this eulogy, I want to thank the
Cyrus family for giving me this opportunity. I am
honored to publicly remember my brother and friend.*

*As each of us looks around this setting and
gathering this afternoon, our first thought may likely
be that the only one missing is Gene. He is not
absent. We are here because Gene Cyrus is very
much a part of each of us. Since we learned of
Gene's diagnosis last September, we all have
struggled in our own way to try to prepare for the
possible loss of this dear son, husband, father,
grandfather, brother, cousin, uncle, nephew, co-
worker, neighbor and friend. And as we read the
journal written faithfully by Judi and the girls, we
could sense the optimism which we all know is so
very much a part of the Cyrus family. Encouragers
that you are, you provided pictures and updates to
help us believe what we hoped and prayed for, that
Gene was going to conquer this horrific assault, this
attack, which we all believed was so unfair and
undeserved. Naturally, we all were viewing this
heartbreaking marathon primarily from our own
perspectives. It was extremely difficult to fathom
that God, our loving God, who loves each of us
beyond measure, could find Gene's suffering
beneficial to a "greater good" or serve the will and
purposes of our Creator. Throughout the past year,
we have wrestled with how to cope with the impact*

of his ordeal and how we might help him and his family conquer this scourge of an enemy. For most of us, it has given us the opportunity to summon from the past the many memories of our experiences with Gene and his family.

To meet Gene Cyrus, it didn't take long, (I'm talking about minutes here, not weeks, months or years) to quickly conclude that your encounter was with a very special person. If you knew a person who had little pretense, it was Gene. If you recalled a co-worker who willingly shared his knowledge and experience to help you learn and progress, it was Gene. If you needed one to trust, it was Gene. If you wanted to liven up a situation and give it a positive spin, you summoned Gene. If you needed a volunteer to help, you called on Gene. If you wanted fun seeking companions to travel with, you called Gene and Judi. If you think of someone selfless and generous beyond measure, you think of Gene. Gene was a "giver" a "sharer," an "encourager" and an employee whose work ethic was a model for all.

I suspect my experiences with Gene Cyrus had many of the same characteristics yours had. I know few, if any, people whose energy level and enthusiasm could top that of Gene's. Cheryl and I first met Gene in 1985 when he and Jaimi arrived ahead of the rest of the family in Stuttgart, Germany where Gene had been recruited by some very astute friends to come to work as a civilian for the Department of the Army. I quickly likened him to one of Winnie the Pooh's best friends and promptly tagged him "Tigger." Tigger roamed the Hundred

Acre Woods with irrepressible good humor singing this song about himself.

"The wonderful things about Tiggers, Tiggers are wonderful things.

Their tops are made outta rubber, and their bottoms are made outta springs.

They're pouncy pouncy bouncy bouncy

Fun Fun Fun Fun Fun

But the most wonderful thing about Tiggers is, I'm the only one."

Gene, like Tigger, was incessantly good humored. He was game to go anywhere, participate in any function and make a positive contribution to every situation.

There was never a quicker mind for puns than Gene's. In almost any normal conversation, Gene would pipe up with a clever pun. If you or someone present responded with one (seldom equal to Gene's) off he'd go, rattling off puns in staccato form. There was none better.

Everyone wanted to be a friend of Gene's, and of course, that was because Gene made everyone feel that he or she was his best friend. They were his. He was there's. I don't recall Gene criticizing a co-worker or anyone else, uh, except for his calling them Dork, Jerk, or some other term of endearment like "Hey, Kid." Gene could and did say things to people, even to superiors, that would have gotten most others fired. He was on safe territory, however, because they knew he was nearly always right, they trusted his opinions, and they knew instinctively that his motives were never self serving or mean spirited. To Gene, his "on target" vocabulary was a teaching aid, and those of us on the receiving end could accept it because we knew that the heart and mind and tongue from whence it came were materials from which saints are made. You just couldn't get angry with Gene. He came across so sincere and honest that you trusted his motives as being good. Gene was transparent and didn't have to have the last word. This was most evident when it came to his real and only true love, Judi.

We all know how Gene would throw out to Judi an idea to go some place or do something that seemed far-fetched or impossible for the average family. Before the two of them were done, the plans were in place and the Cyrus' were off on another adventure that could match or exceed that of Robinson Crusoe. Their propensity to accept and fulfill each other's dreams and challenges is unmatched by any other couple we know. Now, I'd never say all this in the presence of Gene, for fear of his getting the "big head." Can't you just hear his guffaw and "You Dork" and see his big cheesy grin?

If you have ever traveled with Gene and Judi, you know that they can cover more ground and get to the front of the line quicker than any one else. I can't tell you how many times Gene would say, "Come on, lets cross now," and before you could check for on coming traffic, Gene and Judi and the girls would already be on the other side of the street, or when boarding a streetcar, train, or boat, Gene and his family would be on board and seated while we were still trying to get our tickets. And, we were not slackers when it came to covering ground. There was just no way of getting ahead of them.

I really don't know anyone who was more gifted at giving than Gene. It didn't matter where he was or what the item was, he insisted on sharing it with others. You all know how impulsive he was. When he'd see something at the market that excited him (and many items were the source of his excitement), he would say, "Bud, let's get some of these." I'd respond with something like, "What would you do with (and I'd say whatever the excessive amount was). He'd answer, "You and Cheryl can have some, and we'll give the rest away." He wanted others to share his joy and excitement whether it was a place or product or just time.

Gene was one of the luckiest "dudes" (to use one of his phrases) I ever knew. He was one of a group of six guys, five Americans and one German who were known as the Old Farts Ski Club. Several years ago while skiing at Brundage, Idaho, the five of us Americans and another friend decided at the end of a long day to head for home. From where we were, we had to race down a short slope to get sufficient speed to traverse a long flat run. You non-skiers may not know that flat runs are quite tricky because you stay on the bottom of your skis without using the edges for control, except for slight adjustments. Well, Gene went tearing off ahead of the rest of us and was out of sight by virtue of

159

rounding a curve. When we finally rounded the curve and caught up with him, Gene was sprawled out in a snow bank with equipment scattered in every direction. Not wanting us to lose our momentum on the flat, Gene yelled, "I'm OK, keep going. I'll catch up." One of the guys stopped to assist Gene. When the two of them finally caught up with the rest of us, Gene couldn't wait to tell us that his glasses had gone flying, and when he found his glasses, one of the lenses was completely gone. After he had gathered his equipment and prepared to head for the lift, he looked down and there was the lens, completely in tack. It could have happened only to Gene. After a trip to the clinic, Gene learned that he had either broken or nearly broken several ribs. He was unable to ski the rest of the trip, but equally painful was the inability of the "great laugher" to laugh. It is the only time I recall that he had to stifle laughter. It didn't stop his wonderful bushy, bearded grin, however.

When I asked our daughter, Becca, what she remembered most about Gene, here is what she answered, and in the following order:

"He called people, Dork."

"He always had a smile."

"He liked to help plan trips."

"He never said anything out of the way about anyone."

"He supported his girls."

"He truly loved the love of his life, Judi."

"He made everything exciting."

160

"He could eat anything and everything and never gain a pound."

I think she summed up Gene pretty well. Each of you has your own list of who and what Gene was. Each of us will cherish our list and are grateful for it. Each of you could easily use your list for your eulogy of this man. For sure, it would be hard to find something about him that we couldn't share or shouldn't share. In our generation and earlier generations we say he was a "prince of a guy." What a legacy.

I will now read from the book of Revelations, Chapter 20, verses 11 through 15.

11 "Then I saw a great white throne and him who was seated on it. Earth and sky fled from his presence, and there was no place for them. 12 And I saw the dead, great and small, standing before the throne, and books were opened. Another book was opened, which is the Book of Life. The dead were judged according to what they had done as recorded in the books. 13 The sea gave up the dead that were in it, and death and Hades gave up the dead that were in them, and each person was judged according to what he had done. 14 Then death and Hades were thrown into the lake of fire. The lake of fire is the second death. 15 If any one's name was not found written in the Book of Life, he was thrown into the lake of fire."

You may wonder what Gene would say to you today, if he were given that opportunity. I know he

161

would love to see each one of you. For sure he would say, "Don't weep for me." As when he was earth bound, leading the pack, he beat us home. I believe that before he reminisced with you and revisited those many good times of previous days, his first concern for you would be to know whether your name is written in the Lamb's Book of Life, referred to in the book of Revelations. Nothing else would be more important or of greater concern to him. He would beg for you to make certain your name was there along with his and all those who acknowledge that Jesus is the Christ, the Savior and the only way to God the Father. If any of you have never accepted Jesus as your Savior and Lord, acknowledged that his blood covers your every sin and that He is the only way to the Father, it would be Gene's desire and prayer that you make that decision today. There is nothing more important in your life than that one decision.

An unknown person has written:

In the hallways of my memories and the canyons of my heart
I will always remember you!
In the soft snows,
I will always remember you!
In the dawn of spring and dawn of fall,
I will always remember you!
On birthdays, anniversaries and ordinary days,
I will always remember you!
When I am lonely and temped to be bitter,

162

I will always remember you!

When I am disheartened and confused,

I will always remember you!

When good news is too good to keep to myself,

I will always remember you!

In the candlelight of Christmas and in the dawning of Easter,

I will always remember you!

Gene, good buddy, thank you for giving us so much; for helping us along our journey. Life won't be the same without you. Thank you for helping us to be more than we otherwise could have been had you not loved us and invited us along. We know you are waiting with outstretched arms to welcome us when we too will be called home.

THURSDAY, SEPTEMBER 13, 2007

Kalle and I both had a bad day today. Juli reminded us that it was four weeks today. Somehow our unconscious minds must have known that.

This morning I went into the mudroom to clear off the coat rack so the kids could use it. Everything on it was Gene's but when I got to the two old flannel jackets full of burn holes and still smelling a bit like smoke from his burn piles, I lost it. He wore those jackets outside working all the time. I could picture him out there raking stuff into a burn pile then strolling over to sit on the bench by the arena to watch me work with Hope. Now I know why I am having trouble getting myself back

163

to the horses! Even though I always think of them as "my thing", he was always my audience, my cheerleader and my farm hand. I think I am afraid to be out there in the arena and find myself looking for that old blue flannel jacket and it won't be there.

This weeks comfort came in the form of an email from young friend of the family:

Hi Judi, how are you doing?

I meant to send you a message earlier, I guess better late than never. I just wanted to share some random thoughts with you. First I wanted to tell you that I'm amazed at how strong you've been. I know you're hurting and have been through a lot in the last year, but you've handled it all with incredible grace. I really liked the talk you had with the kids during the service. It was sweet and poignant and worked on both a kid level and an adult level.

I've always known Gene as a fun loving, funny guy, but somehow I didn't know about his penchant for puns. He certainly called me a dork many times over the years, but I don't remember him calling me kid. Maybe he reserved that for people his own age or older. Seems like every time I came to visit, the first thing he said to me was "Hey there young man!"

I'll never forget the last time I saw him. After all he'd been through with this terrible disease, he felt he needed to apologize to me. I think because he wasn't feeling well enough to get out of bed and visit with us in the living room that day. But regardless, it just illustrates how he was always more concerned with others than himself, even under the most extreme conditions. I assured him he didn't have to apologize for anything. I wish I would have said more to him that day, but I'm very glad I got the chance to visit with him.

It was good to see all of you recently, although under sad circumstances. God bless you and your family

Nolan

Kalle dreamt about Gene last night. This is her dream:

"I was at a basketball game [Kalle has never been to a basketball game so this was an interesting start] and my daddy came in. He had wings. He asked me if I wanted to go for a ride and I said yes. I had to hold onto his foot so I wouldn't mess up his wings. We were flying over town but his foot was slippery and I was afraid I would fall. He said 'Sorry Kalle, I guess I put too much lotion on my foot.' [also interesting because we had lotioned his feet a lot in the past weeks.] Daddy flew me to Dillon and Ellie's house. Juli wasn't' home, but when Rob saw Dad he got so excited he started to grab him. But Dad said 'Watch out for the wings' and moved out of the way. Rob was jumping so hard he fell off the porch. We watched a movie then Daddy asked me if I wanted a ride home. He flew me home then tucked me in bed and gave me a kiss."

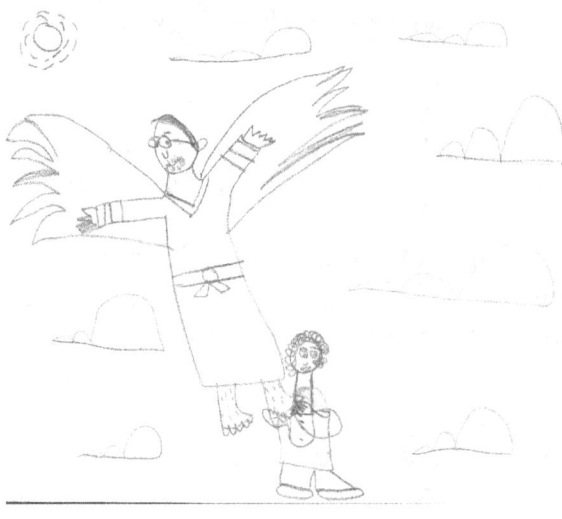

My sister, Bunny, died this morning. She is the one who miraculously survived a burst brain aneurysm, stroke and two brain surgeries last year. She was diagnosed with cancer a few months after Gene. I feel like someone is trying to tell me something. How can it be coincidence that my husband, my dad, and my sister all died in about a month?

I needed some time in the sunshine today, so spent most of the day out at the new (still unfinished) barn. I hiked up on the hill to pick out the spot for Gene's bench. Oh, not sure I mentioned that. We are ordering a granite bench which will have a picture of pine trees with a stream and jumping fish, Gene's name and dates, and a silver picture (the one on the book's cover). We will put it on the new property in the spot I picked out today. That is where his ashes will be placed, along with his journal that people wrote in at the memorial service so we can write our thoughts when we are up there.

Progress is also being made on the memorial garden at church. Thank you everyone who has contributed to that. We hired a landscape designer and he has given us a rough sketch and work is to begin on it around October 5th. Today I ordered a granite stone with Gene's and my dad's names. It will be set into the brickwork under the grape pergola.

It was a beautiful day and I lay on my back in the sun while the tears ran into my ears. I'm sure it won't be the last cry there.

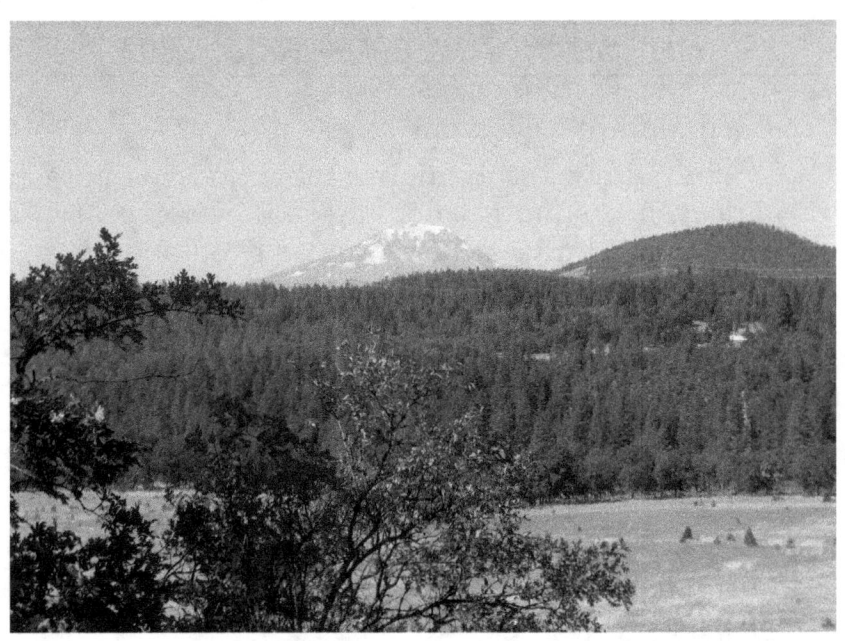

The view from Gene's Garden.

FRIDAY, SEPTEMBER 28, 2007

I got home from Bunny's service in Colorado yesterday. The church was packed with friends and family. The pastor talked about Bunny as a "Prayer Warrior". She had a book that she wrote down the names of people she was praying for. She emailed me last October saying, "I just want you to know that you have always been on my daily prayer list. Of course this will continue. Gene, stay as positive as you can. God will be with you through everything." The subject on her email was "God loves you and so do I." She continued to email words of encouragement until she too became so ill.

THURSDAY, NOVEMBER 15, 2007

Hi Mom, Hi everyone else.

I'm not sure who might still be looking here, but I open it up and get nostalgic on occasion. I miss dad, and I miss all of you - as good as it is to get some stability again, I do miss being "home" so often! And looking at all the pictures - wow, have I had a blessed life with such a great family! I am really looking forward to meeting up with you again in December. Until then, get outside and enjoy the air - winter is here, and at least in this part of the world has brought lots of snow and a welcome crispness and freshness that keeps spirits lively and bright.

love you!

Jaimi

MONDAY, NOVEMBER 19, 2007

Hi Jaimi,

Yeah, I get on occasionally to see if anyone is still visiting too, so it was fun to find your message tonight. I've been thinking about continuing with the "rest of the story" or "road to recovery" but I guess I am still waiting for evidence that there is such a thing. I've been very busy working on the barn and sort of going through the motions of continuing the building of our dreams but other than a bit of satisfaction in seeing jobs done, it kind of seems pointless.

We here are all looking forward to our "run away from Christmas trip" and meeting up with you and Kevin. We miss having you around so much!

Love you! Mom

TUESDAY, NOVEMBER 20, 2007

Hi Mom,

it was nice to see your message! I am glad you are keeping busy and getting at least the satisfaction of jobs done - that is a start and I"m convinced there will be more to come in terms of really feeling happy about it again. I have developed a very bad connection of flying with sadness - every time I get on a plane I close my eyes and relive the past year. Then I end up in Geneva or somewhere for a stupid staff meeting or something and am dysfunctional. I am sure we are on the "road to recovery" but it is not a very straight or even one!

I love you, Mom. Hang in there. And when you get a chance, post some pics of the barn work - I would love to see it

Jaimi

SATURDAY, NOVEMBER 24, 2007
8:12 PM

I had a little trouble getting motivated to work on the barn project, but it is a good distraction now. I work hard all day and it wears me out so I can sleep. I got seven loads of gravel delivered then spread and leveled with Gene's Kubota. I drug in the power poles Rob dropped off to separate the aisle way/stall area from the arena, then compacted all the gravel. In between, I got about 18 tons of hay delivered, most of which the Kubota and I stacked since it was delivered during the week when Rob and Juli were working. I am getting pretty buff!

I got a huge load of steel last week—stall fronts, paddock and arena fencing. It got here in the nick of time cuz then it started snowing and there is no way the trucker could get in and out now! There are piles of panels in front of the barn. My nephew, Cody, and a friend of his drove over from Montana on Thursday and helped me get the stall fronts in, the rubber mats down, and quite a bit of tongue and groove done on the office. They went home yesterday but he is talking about coming back again after Thanksgiving. I got all the insulation done while they were here and Rob put the doors up. The wiring is done in the office and tack room (thanks to Rob and his friend, Jeremy), so now we can actually keep it warm in there! There are still all those panels to put up for paddocks. That could be a nasty job in this weather!

We were all up there today working; Rob and Juli hung sheet rock in the office while I cut the tongue and groove for the stall fronts. I was using a little table saw of my Dad's to rip some of the boards and thinking that it is funny that his daughter is making use of the tools he left behind. I'm sure he is grinning about that. On days that I work up there by myself doing all kinds of two person jobs, I realize that I am a lot like him; no job was ever too big.

Kalle is doing amazingly well. She has sad moments, of course, and cries for her daddy, but she is grieving like a normal person and her behavior has been great. Her teachers even comment on how well she is doing this year. Juli and I had talked about it and decided that Gene must be a lot more persuasive in person and had God working on Kalle. One day she came out of school and said, "Mom, I think I'm healed. I actually feel happy." I told her Juli and I had noticed that and that we think Daddy must have had his talk with God about her. We agreed it is a very special dad who will go all the way to heaven to help his little girl get well.

Jill came home for Thanksgiving. She is doing well in school and has made a nice circle of friends so is not so lonely. We had traditional Thanksgiving dinner and all made it through more or less intact. We are not taking any chances on Christmas though, and are running away to Disney World. Jaimi and Kevin will meet us there. I am not sure if we are cowards or just real smart.

Meanwhile, after feeling like I was pretty tough through Gene's illness, I find that the tears seem to live just behind my eyelids and I begin leaking for any or no reason at all. They say it gets easier with time, but so far it seems to be getting harder; like the reality is setting in that he is not just off on an adventure and will soon be home.

TUESDAY, NOVEMBER 27, 2007

Hurrah! a new journal entry! It is so nice to read and see the update of what you've been doing. What a lot of work for all you guys - makes me wish I was there (ha ha). No really, on the way home from soccer practice today, Kevin made some kind of comment about wanting to take a taxi. I asked him why, and he explained "well, to go to the plane so we can go to Baba and Papa Gene's." It is, of course, perfectly natural to jump in a taxi and head off halfway around the world at any given moment to see the people you love, you know! So we discussed it and concluded that the 3 months since we were last there are simply too long - then counted the days and were happy to see it is only 30 left until we catch up to you on the ship. We also read a book yesterday called "Pony Stories," so are prepping for our next Goldendale visit. So once the barn is done or in between jobs there, I hope you are getting some Hope training time - I believe we have an outstanding plan of a "big horse" ride through the woods!

Love you!

Jaimi

TUESDAY, DECEMBER 04, 2007

Hi Mom,

I'm glad you guys are still using the site, too. I don't get on very often, because, as you know, I like to pretend everything is fine and normal. Reading your journal entries made me tear up a little, though. But then I had to laugh when I read the picture caption about Kevin and Dillon standing "dangerously close to the precarious ugly Christmas tree"!! (O Christmas tree, O Christmas tree, why are you laying on our couch....) And then, I too, got a little nostalgic. I'm sorry that by trying to be "normal", I probably haven't been the best support. But I love you and I am so proud of you, especially for how strong you were through Dad's illness - he needed that!! And now, of course, you need to not be so strong for a little while. Though, I am actually amazed by you, as usual, working so hard on the barn, and planning the memorial for dad and granddad at church. Even in the midst of your grief, you accomplish more than 10 women (or men)! I wish you could take my anatomy final for me. :) Anyway, I miss you, and I am so excited for our trip - remember I am your best travel partner!! (I won't tell jaimi and juli, though.) See you soon! love, Jill

THURSDAY, DECEMBER 13, 2007
11:25 PM

Cody came back for a few more days after Thanksgiving, bringing along his girl friend, my sister, Norma (his mom) and my mom. Cody slaved away at the barn, getting the rest of the tongue and groove on the walls in the breezeway and making a good start on the deck railing for the "Margarita Bar" (observation deck above the office). Norma and I got the posts up for the pergola at the church and also got the walls done in the tack room and tractor bay. So a busy few days.

Last weekend Kalle and I flew to Minnesota to visit Gene's parents. I was a little apprehensive because I have been such a weeper lately and I was afraid I would be a blubbering idiot and just make them feel worse. But it was a great weekend. We had a good visit and of course reminisced about how much Gene meant to all of us. Gene's brother, Larry , two of his sons, Gene's fave auntie Jo, and her daughter, Shannon with two of her sons all

173

came to visit while I was there so all in all a very great weekend.

In the plane coming home, I was hit by a memory of a trip we made and could not get seats together. He was sitting about ten rows ahead of me. When the beverage service started, the flight attendant brought me a glass of champagne with a sort of apologetic explanation that it was sent by the gentleman in 14C. Gene thought he was pretty funny acting like a smitten stranger.

When we drove in the driveway, I asked Kalle if she was glad to be home. She said, "yes but I will miss Gramma and Grampa. What if they need help around the house?" I'm not sure what she did to help but she WAS good company and a very good traveling companion (Jill, you have competition!)

Rob has nearly finished the office at the barn. I went up yesterday and got some of the T&G done on the ceiling. Nearly killed myself getting the 12 foot boards up over my head and screwing them on. When Rob got there he fixed all of my mistakes. I agreed to do something less critical today so went and worked on the pergola at church. One more afternoon should finish the trim and it will be complete except for the grape vines, which I plan to dig up from my dad's garden in the Spring. Tonight Rob finished the ceiling so now the office is ready for sealer/paint. Then flooring and trim!

I've felt pretty good this week. It has been busy with projects during the day and kids Christmas programs in the evenings. Next week is Ellie's birthday and then we head out for Disneyworld. We are excited about the trip and also about seeing Jaimi and Kevin. We have not seen Kevin for five months now. We got kind of used to

174

having him around more! Oh yeah, and Jaimi too (Love you, Jaimi!) though it has only been 3 months since we saw her.

Gene's sis, Leslie, sent Juli a Christmas card noting how much Gene always loved Christmas and that he was probably searching out the best tree ever. Made me feel a little guilty that we are not even putting up a tree. Dillon did hang some paper ornaments on a house plant, though. At least it won't fall over.

From the Guest Book:

WEDNESDAY, DECEMBER 19, 2007

It's good you've kept this up. Just want you to know that I think a lot about you all and Gene. Got a little ditty for you.

The First Christmas
The first Christmas came and we still had our tears.
Our Papa, Son, Brother, Husband and Friend
Was no longer here to spread the good cheer.
They say life goes on
You have to get back in the game
But with memories so fresh
Christmas can't be the same.
He was such a bright light
Especially around this time of year.
He would giggle and cackle
And remind us all it was here.
The twinkle in his eyes
And that confident walk
The way he could get anybody to talk
That incredible enthusiasm for all that is life
The love that he had for his kids and his wife.

175

So Christmas isn't the same this year.
Down here anyway.
But I imagine up in heaven
It'll be livelier that day.
Gene will be next to Jesus
Eating Christmas dinner with a fork.
And Jesus will be mighty surprised
At the first Angel to call him Dork!
Best wishes – Big Al

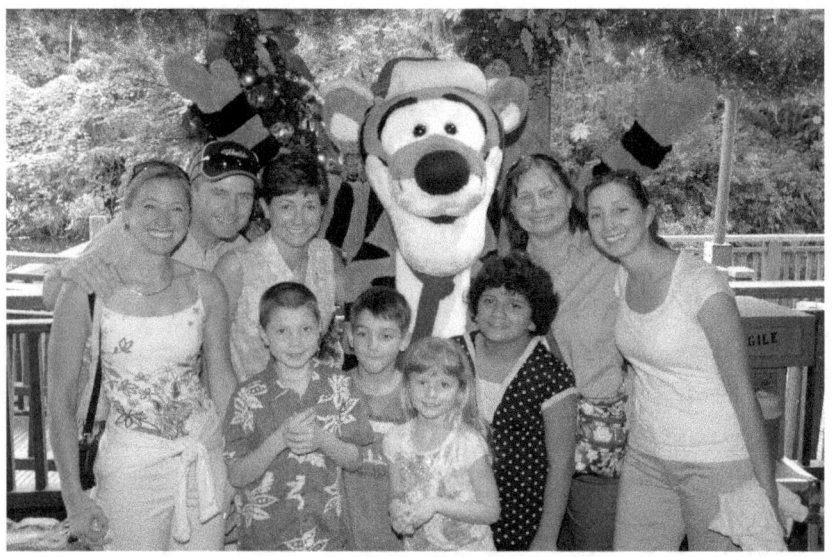

Tigger will always be with us.

SATURDAY, JANUARY 05, 2008

I am having a lonely day. I had no idea how much I would miss him! I have lost all joy in the things I used to love. People wish for us a "happy new year" or a "better year this year" but I can't imagine how it can ever be better. He won't be coming back this year. None of the broken things in my life will go away.

I'm sorry I took him for granted. I hope it's true that he is in a better place now, but he loved life here so much, even with all the problems, it is almost as hard for me to imagine a better place for him as it is hard to image a "better year" for me.

I hope he knows how much I love him. I wish I had been better at showing him.

MONDAY, JANUARY 07, 2008
10:34 AM

I just checked in today feeling a little blue and was so happy to find messages from Leslie, Al and Heather. Al, it's been a long time and I so much appreciate your ditty. You have kept us in giggles and tears for the past year. I wish we could roll back the clock to last year's Christmas poem when we still believed in a win.

We all made it home safely from a different than we planned kind of vacation in Florida. To make a long story short, we were not allowed to board the cruise ship because Dillon had been sick the night before. If you ever go on a cruise and get asked if anyone has vomited, had diarrhea, coughing or sneezing in the past 48 hours, YOU MUST LIE. They did not even check Dillon or acknowledge that he was definitely not sick when we arrived at the port (running all over the terminal playing with the other kids) but because we truthfully answered "yes" to the question, we were denied boarding. Disney Cruise Line does not have an alternate plan for guests they turn away, so we ended up spending most of the day trying to find rooms to stay in. We were very frustrated and upset about the whole thing, partly, as Jill pointed out, because we felt like we had so little control over what was happening to us, which is pretty much how we have felt for the past year. There was nothing available on Disney property and we ended up staying in an off-resort (non-Disney) hotel then taking inconvenient transportation to spend way too much time in over-crowded Disney parks. Not what we had hoped for our vacation, but we were together and we were NOT here so at least those two goals were accomplished.

Now I am trying to get some kind of a refund for the cruise. Can you believe they said we could not get a refund when they denied boarding!!!!!????? They said we would need to submit a claim to the insurance, but the insurance says that since we didn't have certification of illness from a doctor, they don't pay. Since Dillon was no longer sick, that would have been a bit hard to get even if they HAD let us see the ship doctor, which we demanded but were also denied!

So lots to do but most of it not fun. So off I go.

THURSDAY, JANUARY 10, 2008
10:39 AM

Today's photo is actually a Christmas card from my brother, George. I modified his card to put the "In loving memory: Lloyd Johnson, Gene Cyrus, Bunny Rohrig" message on the front instead of the inside where you wouldn't see it.

George used to make a Christmas card every year but a few years ago decided not to do it anymore. We all used to wait anxiously for his card to arrive so have been giving him heck about not making them. He said he ran out of ideas, which I don't believe for a minute! So I was surprised when I opened this card and it brings tears to my eyes each time I look at it. Sometimes I feel very alone in my grief and loneliness and this is a reminder of how much other people in my life hurt with me.

I asked George for permission to post it on this site because I thought it might touch many of you as well.

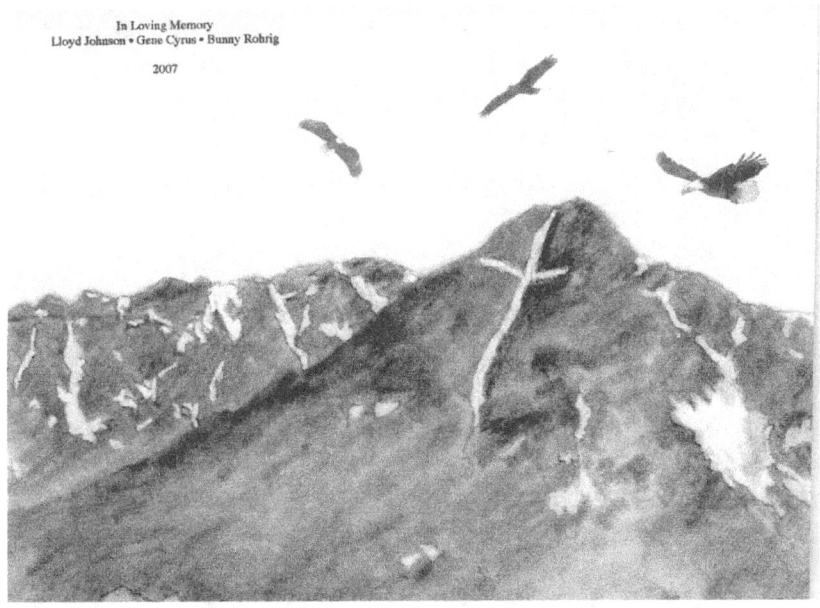

In Loving Memory
Lloyd Johnson • Gene Cyrus • Bunny Rohrig

2007

WEDNESDAY, JANUARY 23, 2008

I have been reading a new book called, "Getting to the Other Side of Grief." This is a pretty good book, written by a counselor and a pastor, who have each lost their spouses. I like it because it gives you specific tasks to do to help you work through the grief process. I find I am guilty of trying to run away and trying to deny or stifle my feelings, thinking I am just dwelling on my sadness and making it worse. But they say you have to let yourself grieve, and in fact work at it, or it will never really heal.

So assignment number one: What do I miss most about Gene?

I think I most miss seeing him work around the place while I played with the horses. I miss joking with him about how living my dream is a lot of work for him, and calling ourselves the little farmer couple. I also miss just being with him, especially driving Kalle back and forth to school and I miss meeting the smile in his eyes over the top of her head when she says something funny (which is often!) or profound.

What do I wish he had said or done?

I wish that he had left me a letter. I helped him write letters to the grandkids and when he asked if I needed one, I told him that I didn't because I knew how he felt about me. As his mom says, he had me on such a high pedestal that if I ever fell off, I would break my leg. But now I wish I had a letter to find when I am searching for keepsakes and memories.

Did I mention I also do the search thing at my dad's house? It has not sold yet, so I go over fairly often to check on things and I find myself leafing through books and going through cupboards looking for mementos. This week I found a letter he had written us with his death instructions. I had not found anything like this printed out, not with his will or the trust papers. But I found it on the old computer he had given Kalle. It says he wants his ashes sprinkled at Rifle Falls. I had no idea. But he said he always had good memories of there and it made me think of him taking us fishing there when we were little.

MONDAY, JANUARY 28, 2008

It has snowed a lot here in the past few days. More than I have ever seen at once here. I just came in from my morning trudge around feeding the horses. I cut back towards the house behind the aviaries. Oh yeah, did I mention the snow collapsed the aviaries so now that is another big Spring cleanup job. Anyway, this brought me by the bench Gene gave me for our 33rd anniversary. It was covered with snow, so I brushed it off, thinking of how surprised and happy I was when he gave it to me. If I think of memories of when I felt especially touched by his love, this is one of them.

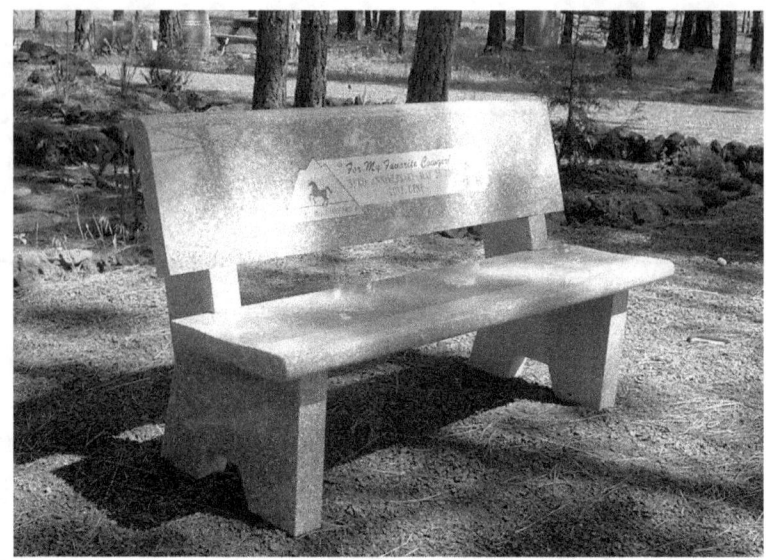

Another was one time when we lived in Preston and I was having such a bad day that I "ran away" and ended up parking the car by the gate on the other side of the DNR land next to our place. I walked into the woods along the horse super highways Gene had painstakingly cut all around through the undergrowth so that I would have riding trails. Seeing all that work he had done just for me. . . Well, right up there in the top memories.

When I try to think of really great things I did to reciprocate, I come up short. I guess I am not really a romantic. I thought I showed him every day that I loved him by fixing his favorite meals or whatever, but it sure doesn't have the same impact. I took what we had for granted; I always assumed we would grow old together and I pictured us sitting on the porch enjoying the sunsets.

I did try to shower Gene with love during his illness. I actually loved taking care of him. I miss driving him to his doctor's appointments and

182

holding his hand while we said bedtime prayers together. I miss reading him to sleep at night. I even miss lifting him in and out of his wheelchair and taking care of his hygiene. He often asked me "if it was all too much" for me but I hope I convinced him that it was my privilege to take care of him. It gave me the chance to show him how I felt.

I have been reading a book called, "Praying to the God You Can Trust" by Leith Anderson. The tagline on the cover is, "There is hope even when God says no to your prayers." Anderson quotes 1 John 5:14: "This is the confidence we have in approaching God: that if we ask anything according to His will, he hears us." He proceeds to give all kinds of examples of why it might not be God's will to say "yes" to all prayers, but even when the answer is "no", God is in control and has a plan beyond our comprehension. Anderson also says that it is best to try to understand God's will and then ask for favors, since obviously that ups the chances for a "yes" answer.

I have been struggling to understand God's plan, understand his "no" answer to all the prayers begging for Gene's life, and all the seemingly "no" answers to my prayers for comfort since his death and what His will is for my life now that it seems so empty. One of the biggest "emptinesses" for me is that I have regrets about how we spent some of the last years of Gene's life. We had so many problems with our adopted six-pack that I changed to a person I did not really like. I was angry all the time; I took their rejection of and anger at me personally and I lashed back at them. I resented the constraints their actions put on our lives as we gave them 24/7 supervision to protect them from doing things that hurt others or put them at risk. And now I feel guilty for convincing Gene we should take on that burden and for not being the fun, joyous companion he married during the past hard years.

It seems grossly unfair that we would struggle for years with the kids and then nearly on the eve of their all leaving home, I would lose Gene. The other night I prayed to understand God's will for my life, why he would take my husband just when we neared a time when we could put our lives back on a happier track. And I prayed that Gene understood my sorrow and contrition for not handling the issues better, for letting them get in the way of our own relationship. I prayed that he knew how much I loved him in spite of my actions and that he still loved me too.

The next day I received a phone call from Jaimi saying she had been thinking about her dad and how much he loved me. That growing up in that love was such a privilege. I got teary and couldn't tell her how much this meant to me so later I emailed her to tell her she had answered a prayer with her phone call. Later she emailed me:

"I was so happy to read your message this morning - well, happy and sad. First, sad that you have been struggling with some very tough and complex emotions and that I'm not able to help you through it. I like to think that I can understand some of what you're feeling, but don't really know if I do. I do know that we Cyrus ladies have a tendency to take too much self-responsibility for things beyond our control, and to criticize ourselves (our actions, our feelings, our behavior) much more than the world

around us does. I also know that this holds true for you and for Dad.; The past years were extremely tough, and you were not the person you wanted to be. And not the person Dad fell in love with many years ago. That does not mean, however, that he lost that love for you! You were still there, even if often masked by stress and anger - when those things fell away, you were your real you again. Many times, also in the past couple of years, we would all be sitting at the table playing silly games after dinner, making jokes and telling silly stories, and just like always, Dad's eyes would shine while bantering with his "Beaner".

Mom, he loved you so much! Despite the trouble in your lives, you both are still an inspiration to me. And how you loved each other and cared for each other (him helping you realize your dreams, you inspiring him in the earlier days and then caring heart and soul for him when he needed it most) is a legacy that most of us can only dream to experience. Things don't have to be perfect to be exceptional.

If you fell off a pedestal, maybe it was just time for it to go away. Life is easier if we live it on the ground. You are great for who you are and what you give to all those around you - and you don't need a pedestal to be great. You just are. I remember you helping Dad onto the couch one day last summer, and he looked up at you like you were the only woman in the world. As sad as sometimes watching him made me in those days, that was a beautiful moment that is imprinted on my brain forever.

185

I hope I haven't made you lose it again. But if I did, then just lose it for a while. Have a good cry, and then go out and rake some pine needles, breathe deeply some fresh air, and smile a bit that you are so loved and cherished. Not only by Dad - you have a lot of fans out here. :)

I love you mom.
Jaimi"

Jaimi's message was an answer to my prayer. And I understand that God's will is that I feel loved.

I have learned that loss is even harder when there are unspoken words or unresolved issues in a relationship that ends in death. I touched on these feelings with Gene before he died, but we did not have a real in-depth discussion because as Gene hung onto his hope for a miracle, he also lived somewhat in denial of his impending death. This made it hard to have "last conversations."

SIX MONTHS LATER

Juli told me yesterday that she wakes up every morning thinking about her dad. But she thinks of him as he was at the end of his life and she worries because he always said that was not how he wanted to be remembered. I told her I wake up every morning with the same thoughts. I think it is because it was such a momentous time in our lives that it overshadows everything else that ever happened. But that is kind of sad. We are going to start watching videos from earlier days and trying to refix our thoughts on who he was throughout his life.

I also have the sadness of reliving his death over and over. I have not talked a lot about it, and I hesitate to detail that time here, it is so private and personal, but I wish I had known what it would be like to be with him when he died. It might have made it easier for me to know I was doing the right things. So in case you are going through a trial like this, I will share this night of my life.

The tumor in Gene's back started hurting badly again the day before he died so I increased his pain medication. He slept most of the day. I helped him wash and clean his teeth about 8:30 and tucked him into bed. Juli kissed him good-night and they went home. I got ready for bed and we said our prayers. Gene was concerned about praying for my dad. I read for awhile and then crawled into bed and went to sleep. I woke up about 1:00 because Gene was moaning loudly. I gave him some pain medication and sat by him for a few minutes, then went back to bed. A couple hours later we repeated this. Gene did not really wake up either time, but I knew he was in pain because he was moaning loudly. About 4:30 I woke up again. He was moaning loudly and breathing very hard, like he was struggling to breathe, taking big but quick gasping breaths. I gave him more pain medication, then sat on the chair beside his bed. He was lying on his left side so I sat on the left side of the bed and held his left hand. He usually calmed if I would hold and stroke his hand, so this is what I did. By now he was mumbling some, but not looking at me and I am not sure he even knew I was there. He looked towards the ceiling and

187

reached out (towards the ceiling, not towards me) and said, "Help me, help me." I don't think he was talking to me. I think he was seeing someone else and calling for their help. At the time, I thought my dad must have died and that Gene was calling to him. But my dad lived two more days, so that was probably not who he saw. Then he mumbled, "I love you." Again, I don't think he was talking to me. I administered more pain medication and decided that if he didn't seem better by 5:00, I would call hospice to see if I should give him something else. At 4:58, as I sat beside him holding his hand, his eyes defocused and he went still and quiet.

I called hospice and told the nurse he had died. About 5:30 I called Juli and Rob to tell them. I did not want to wake them up, knowing they would need their energy to get through this day, but needed to call before Rob went to work so he would be there. About a half hour later, Juli got here and said good-bye to her dad. Kalle woke up about 6:30. At first I did not want to tell her until Colleen (the hospice nurse) got there, but decided, as usual, not to let her perceive it on her own. So I sat down with her and told her Daddy had died. She was very calm and went in to see him and kissed him good-bye.

It took about 90 minutes for hospice to get there because they are based in The Dalles. I sat beside Gene but didn't really know what to do. I wish I had taken this time to talk to him in case his soul was still lingering but I did not think of that. I wish I had dressed him, but I did not think of that. I think if Colleen (our hospice nurse) had come, she would have helped me do these things, but she was not available and a nurse I did not know came. She checked Gene, called the funeral home, removed some of the hospice loaner items and emptied drug containers. She did not know us and we did not know her and I think she sensed that it would not be helpful for her to try to do anything personal for us. Thankfully, Cathleen, the chaplain who we had been working with, came with her. After Rob, Dillon and Ellie arrived, Cathleen led us in prayer around Gene's bed. This was a very good thing to do and I so appreciate that she thought to lead us in this way. She held one of Gene's hands, told him good-bye and helped us all say good-bye.

The funeral home arrived then so we went to sit in the living room, not wanting to watch them move Gene's body. When Kalle understood they were here to take his body away, she got upset and ran upstairs. I followed her and sat with her there, deciding it would be better if she did not watch them take him out of the house. I talked to her about Daddy's soul being gone from his body and that it wasn't really him they were taking away. I reminded her that he was in heaven now and that his body did not hurt him anymore and that he did not live in the sick body anymore. She calmed down and was a champ the rest of the day.

If you expect to lose someone you love, as macabre as this sounds, it would be good to plan ahead for what you want to do. In those moments, we were not thinking very well and it would have been better if we had had a plan. And I should have been prepared for the fact that Colleen might not be the one to come. I had a very hard time when I saw a strange nurse get out of the car. We were very fortunate that we also had a relationship with Cathleen so we did not feel as alone as we would have otherwise.

I am writing these last entries, not part of the Caring Bridge journal, but rather from my personal journal and also things I think I need to share. I consider that if you are reading this, you have probably lost someone you love and are looking for answers to why did this happen and how do you get through it. Those are the answers I am looking for, too. I did tell you that I don't really have any answers for you, but I have done a lot of reading and find that the stories that help me most are those of others who have been down this road. I appreciate hearing that they had some of the same feelings and reactions as me because it helps me realize I am not crazy. I hope that if they got through this, maybe I can too.

I am still shocked that I was so strong all through Gene's illness and even for awhile after his death. It is now nearly six months since he died and I feel worse now than I did then. But in the book I just read, "Getting to the Other Side of Grief" the author tells how she hit bottom about five months after her husband's death and then realized she would have to go to work to get through the grief. This encouraged me that because I seem to be getting sadder and more discouraged does not mean I will never get better. I am now embarked on executing the tasks in the book. Today I filled a box with the precious mementos I want to keep; silly things like his glasses, comb and favorite stuffed Moose, Mayfield, practical things like his wallet, Swiss Army knife and hunting knife, and touching things like cards the girls have made for him through the years and all the semi-X-rated pictures of me I found in his desk drawer. I put the box on the floor in my closet, so it is there when I need it, but the things are not where I will run across them every day.

The book talks about taking off wedding rings and says that needs to be done because I am not married anymore. I still feel married though, so the rings stay on. Maybe someday I can face that, but not right now. Maybe never. We were married for 37 years; it is not easy to move away from that

I feel very alone. Juli, Rob, Dillon and Ellie are all with me. I talk to Jill on the phone every day and Jaimi every week. I will see Jaimi this weekend as she will be in the US on business and will make a stopover in Portland to meet us. We all talk about how much we miss their dad, but I don't want to put my grief on top of their own, so for the most part, I try to laugh and talk and go on about life as normally as possible. Of course I am not fooling them, but I do my best. Writing this, sharing my story, is my way of finding a friend to share my grief. I hope in some way, knowing that you are not alone in your grief, will help you too.

NINE MONTHS LATER

In April, I flew to Germany to stay with Kevin while Jaimi made a business trip to Portugal. It was a rare and precious treat to have him all to myself. I walked to school with him as he zoomed along on his scooter, then met him after school for the walk home. We played basketball on the school playground and soccer in the park. I even got to be his parent proxy at a parents' breakfast at his after school program.

But in the midst of all the fun, I woke up one night sobbing from my first dream about Gene. I had dreamt that I was working on the yard at church. Gene drove up to see if I was ready to go home. I asked him to go pick up some supplies I needed and he acted grumpy with me, then started driving off. As he drove away, I saw a woman was sitting next to him. I ran after him to see who it was. When I asked him, he got angry and told me he had wanted a divorce for the last year and a half. I started crying and woke up with my face covered in tears and crying out loud. I felt bad all day, and in fact the rest of the trip. On the airplane ride home I kept finding my face wet with tears, just leaking out of my eyes.

Trying to make some sense out of it, I shared this dream with Colleen, Gene's hospice nurse. This was her response:

"I am sorry about Gene's message. I agree with Jill [who told me he was telling me to get on with my life], *and would go further to say that Gene knew how to get your attention. If it was a simple "permission to get on with your life", you would've blown it off. What little I knew of Gene, it wasn't meant to be mean, rather, it was a heartbreaking, selfless gesture! He wanted you to sit up and pay attention to the heart of the message, and not the details…he may be telling you to let go of his hand, so you can grasp another's."*

In thinking more about it, the "year and a half" prior to the dream led back nearly exactly to the day we learned that Gene had cancer.

In any case, the tears continued and I finally broke down and saw our family doctor for a prescription for antidepressants. I had tried to avoid this because the books I was reading told me it was better to feel and deal with the grief rather than masking it. I now disagree with this advice; only after getting on antidepressants was I able to begin to see myself as still having some kind of life before me.

TEN MONTHS LATER

On our way to church on Father's Day, Kalle said it wasn't a very good day because she did not have a father. I told her of course she did; that her daddy would always be her father even if he wasn't on earth anymore. So she asked what we would do to celebrate Father's Day. We decided it would be great to hang the bird houses painted at Gene's memorial service in his garden as our Father's Day tribute.

Lately I have found myself better able to get through each day, and even began to get more motivated about working on projects or with my horses. But I still did not really see myself in the future. I was going through each day as it needed going through but really had no long term outlook for my life.

So I decided to start working on house plans for the new property. Of course this house could not be built until the one I live in sold, but it was a forward looking project and that seemed like a good idea. I bought lots of house plan books but could not really find one that satisfied my criteria for a very special house with specific spaces but restricted size (I wanted to build something smaller than the house I am in). Finally I called on my friend, John, who designed our church to see if he might be interested in helping me. I emailed him and that very day he called to talk to me about it. He said he assumed it was something I wanted to do right away. I explained that it was not really time critical since I couldn't build it now anyway but that it was more a "mind changing" project. He said, "Well, I really would like to help you with it. . ." and I waited for the but, ". . . in fact, so much so that I was thinking of coming over this weekend."

John came over the next Friday. We sat on the hillside at the house site with a picnic lunch, enjoyed the view, and talked about Gene and how hard losing him was. John said, "I can't imagine what I would do if I lost my wife." I told him he was right. You absolutely can't imagine in your wildest imaginings what it is like to lose your life partner. And I, at least, had no clue how badly I would handle it. I felt so strong during his illness that I was convinced I would just continue plowing on after he was gone. It wasn't like that at all!

We spent the next couple of months working on house plans. John made a couple of trips here and I made one to the west side to visit his family. We came up with a very exciting plan. One day I put on some music then went into my office to do some correspondence. I couldn't hear the music and thought that in my new house, the office would be right off of the living room so I would be able to hear the music. At that moment, I realized this was the first vision I had had of myself actually living in the future.

I still have not sold my house so have not built the new one but John gave me a much bigger gift than some really awesome house plans; he gave me my life back.

ONE YEAR LATER

Jaimi and Kevin arrived on August 3 for a 3 week visit. It is the first time we have all been together since the month before Gene died (all but Kevin were here for the memorial service). So rather than ignoring the elephant in the room, we decided to commemorate the anniversary of his death by spreading his ashes at "Papa Gene's Garden" at the new property.

Of course the occasion called for a champagne toast to the man we all miss so much, then we each shared a favorite memory about Gene. Kevin told how much he liked wrestling with Papa Gene; Dillon and Rob love to remember how whenever they came in the door he would call out in his big voice, "Hello, Mr. Dillon. Hello, Mr. Rob!" Kalle told a memory of when he first took her to Kindergarten she was nervous so she took off his glasses and rubbed his eyes as she loved to do (she always stroked his eyes or my hair for security). A boy next to her said, "what is she doing?" and her dad said, "playing with my eyes" like it was the expected behavior for a new school girl. He always made her feel accepted, loved and normal. Jill remembered how when she wrecked the Mercedes (Jaimi brags that she is the only one of us who never wrecked it), he just clicked his tongue in disgust, but the next day he sent her flowers because he felt bad for being mad at her. Jaimi remembered how, as a 12 year old, she went with him ahead of the rest of us on the move to Germany and he would wake her up every morning so she could tell him which tie he should wear. Juli remembered how he DIDN'T send her flowers when she wrecked the Mercedes (I didn't get flowers either time I wrecked it) And my favorite memory was of him cutting miles of trails through the woods in Preston so I could ride my horses.

EPILOGUE

It has now been 18 months since Gene died. I still feel very alone at times. One of the worst times for me are at night in my lonely bed. I did make it easier this winter by buying a heated mattress pad so at least I could crawl into a warm bed instead of an icy cold one. The other times that are hard for me, embarrassingly, have to do with work and responsibility. There is so much work to do to keep this place up and the animals tended and many days I find myself sobbing because I have to do it all alone. Yesterday I had to clean up the mess created by a hay tent that was crushed under the snow this winter. As I was doing it, I was thinking about a few years ago when our neighbors' RV tent suffered the same fate. Gene and I went over and cleaned it up together because our neighbor has emphysema and couldn't do it. Now here I was repeating the task. But alone. I also feel alone and overwhelmed sometimes by responsibility for making decisions like "repair or replace the roof" (I replaced it), "trade in for a cheaper car?" (so far I haven't), "blow money on a family vacation for Christmas or be responsible about the diminishing funds?" (I blew it), etc.

But now I also have many good days when I feel capable and alive. I actually started internet dating and am quite thrilled with myself for being so adventurous. I have to say, the first date went badly. Since I was only 17 when we got married, I can't say I ever had a LOT of experience dating. And of course that was nearly forty years ago. So this was pretty new territory. On the first date (lunch with a very nice man) I was so uncomfortable that after we parted ways I called Juli and told her that when I got to heaven I was going to kill her dad for putting me through this. I never heard from that poor guy again, but did come up with a couple more "boyfriends" whose company I have enjoyed. For awhile I was quite the social butterfly, getting ready for my Friday night dates and getting lots of phone calls. Rob told Juli it was like living with a fifty year old teenager. Things have kind of settled down now. I am seeing one man with some regularity and we are talking about whether we are right for each other in a permanent sense.

Kalle continues to have occasional vivid dreams about her dad. Recently, after a particularly bad fight with me, Kalle had this dream:

"It was after supper and I went upstairs. Daddy was up there doing some work and said, "Hi, Little Mouse" when he saw me. I said Hi and asked him if he wanted to wrestle. He said sure so we wrestled for awhile. Then he flew out the window. I went and looked out and saw he was down working in the garden so I went down and helped him for awhile. Then he said he had to go and told me, "Be nice to your mom. Remember what I told you".

This was not the first time she had a dream where he gave her advice about her relationship with me. I am grateful for his help! But I still have never had another dream.

Kalle has come to accept us as a twosome. Recently she drew these pictures of her family.

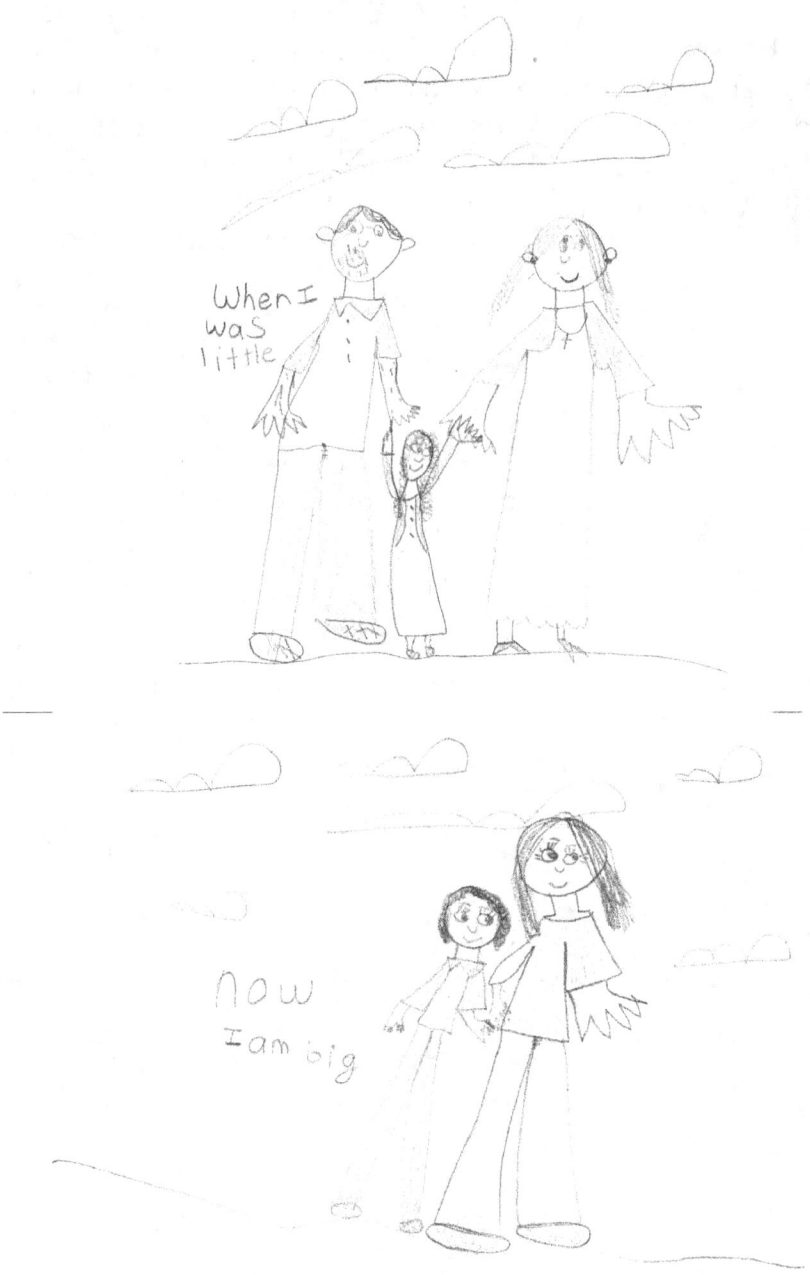

When I
was
little

now
I am big

I think often of Gene's favorite inspiration, "The Station". It seems that life does go on. I will never stop missing Gene but finally, at least most days, I am continuing on the journey without him. I wonder, when I hear that whistle blowing for my final station, will he be waiting there on the platform, waving, anxious to welcome me home?

Acknowledgments

Thanks to all who followed our journey in person or via the Caring Bridge site. Thanks to contributors to this work including our Guestbook visitors, especially Big Al who provided all with many laughs and tears along the way, and to my daughters and fellow journal authors Juli, Jaimi and Jillian.

Special thanks also go to Jaimi, who, even though living in Germany, managed to be with us through this entire journey, often in person but always in spirit.

Kudos to Jillian for accepting the challenge to head off to school, at a time when it was so hard to leave.

And thanks to Juli, Rob, Dillon and Ellie for helping Kalle through the dark tunnel of loss.

www.ingramcontent.com/pod-product-compliance
Lightning Source LLC
Chambersburg PA
CBHW070840310526
45793CB00010B/90